D1276107

Seth Hardcastle was breathtaking sex on legs, and trouble and heartache.

And she'd had more than enough trouble and heartache to last her a lifetime.

But not enough breathtaking sex, her body whispered. No, she wasn't even going to speculate about what sex with Seth would be like, and quickly she eased her fingers free from his, praying her cheeks weren't as red as they felt.

'I really must go,' she said, backing up a step.

'I must, too,' he replied, not moving at all.

'I'll see you tomorrow, then,' she mumbled, and he nodded, and she walked briskly down the corridor.

I am not going to look back, she told herself. *Looking back is what teenagers do when they're desperate to know whether the boy they're interested in might be interested in them, so I'm not going to look back.*

But she did.

A&E DRAMA

Blood pressure is high and pulses are racing in these fast-paced, dramatic stories from Mills & Boon® Medical Romance™. They'll move a mountain to save a life in an emergency, be they the crash team, ER doctors, fire, air and land rescue, or paramedics. There are lots of critical engagements amongst the high tensions and emotional passions in these exciting stories of lives and loves at risk!

A&E DRAMA

Hearts are racing!

Recent titles by the same author:

THE PLAYBOY CONSULTANT*
THE SURGEON'S MARRIAGE*
DOCTOR AND SON*

The Baby Doctors trilogy

Maggie Kingsley returns to the Belfield Infirmary with this sparkling story of doctors at work…and in love!

THE SURGEON'S MARRIAGE DEMAND

BY
MAGGIE KINGSLEY

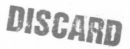
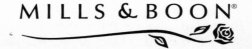

For my mother, who's always been there for me
through the good times and the bad.

*MILLS & BOON and
MILLS & BOON with the Rose Device
are registered trademarks of the publisher.*

*First published in Great Britain 2004
Large Print edition 2005
Harlequin Mills & Boon Limited,
Eton House, 18-24 Paradise Road,
Richmond, Surrey TW9 1SR*

© Maggie Kingsley 2004

ISBN 0 263 18453 6

*Set in Times Roman 16 on 17 pt.
17-0305-55138*

*Printed and bound in Great Britain
by Antony Rowe Ltd, Chippenham, Wiltshire*

CHAPTER ONE

DEBORAH would have said she was crazy. Deborah would have taken one look at the peeling paintwork, the worn and scruffy floor of the waiting room of the Belfield Infirmary's A and E department, and said, 'Liv, are you out of your mind?'

A small smile curved Olivia's lips. Maybe her sister was right. Maybe she *was* crazy, but this was what she wanted. Not a pristine, state-of-the-art A and E department, but a place that needed her as much as she needed it. A department where all her organisational talents could be used to the full. She couldn't wait to get started.

'They're moving very quickly today, aren't they?'

Olivia turned in her seat to see an elderly woman smiling at her, and smiled back. 'Quickly?' she repeated.

The woman nodded. 'Madge on Reception said she didn't think I'd have to wait for more than two hours today.'

Olivia's smile vanished. Two *hours*? OK, so the waiting room was crowded but according to the head of human resources the department had two consultants, a specialist registrar, a junior doctor, plus a full complement of nurses. If they couldn't manage a fast turnaround on a wet Sunday afternoon in September, how on earth did they manage at Christmas, New Year and during the summer holidays?

'What are you here for, dear, if you don't mind me asking?' the woman continued, and Olivia coloured guiltily.

'Stomach pains,' she muttered, and the woman tutted sympathetically, which made Olivia feel even guiltier, but she could hardly tell her elderly companion the truth. That she was snooping. Snooping to find out how efficient—or otherwise—the Belfield's A and E department might be.

It had been her sister Deborah's idea.

'Why don't you turn up incognito before you officially start work?' she'd said when Olivia had told her she'd got the job. 'It's amazing what you can find out when nobody knows who you are.'

Her sister had been right. Of course, her sister had also said Olivia would be married with a family by the time she was thirty, but big sisters couldn't be right about everything. Not even big sisters who had the perfect job, the perfect husband and two equally perfect children.

Unconsciously Olivia shook her head. It wasn't Deborah's fault that everything she touched turned to gold, whereas she always seemed to end up with the fuzzy side of the lollipop. And things were going to be different from now on. As from tomorrow she was the new clinical director in charge of the A and E department of the Belfield Infirmary, and it sounded good. Actually, it sounded downright wonderful.

'Uh-oh, looks like trouble,' the elderly woman beside her exclaimed.

It did. Olivia had noticed the two young men earlier. One was clearly in need of medical attention while the other was obviously only there for moral support. Unfortunately his idea of moral support had been to sing raucous football songs and drink from a bottle for the last forty minutes, but up until now he'd simply been an irritant. Now he'd obviously become bored with waiting and had lurched across to the reception desk. Judging by the receptionist's tight expression, he wasn't engaging in pleasantries.

An uneasy frown creased Olivia's forehead as she watched him. Situations like this could all too easily get out of hand, and whatever the receptionist was saying wasn't working. Neither, it appeared, was her panic button if the non-arrival of any burly security men was anything to go by.

Oh, blow the incognito bit, Olivia decided, getting quickly to her feet. The receptionist needed help, and she needed it now. But before she could move, her elderly companion reached up and caught hold of her arm.

'It's all right, dear,' she said as the door leading to the examination rooms suddenly opened. 'Mr Hardcastle's here. He'll soon sort everything out.'

Olivia turned in the direction of her companion's gaze, and blinked. So this was Seth Hardcastle. Seth Hardcastle who, according to his file, was thirty-six, single and one of A and E's two consultants. What the file had failed to mention—and Olivia really felt it should have—was that he was also six feet two, with thick black hair and possessed a pair of the bluest eyes she'd ever seen.

'He's very good looking, isn't he?' her companion whispered.

He was. He also looked like the kind of man Olivia had spent a lifetime avoiding. The kind of man whose idea of commitment was a long weekend. The kind of man who'd broken more female hearts than she'd had *caffe lattes.* She sat down again fast.

'He's actually a real sweetie underneath,' the elderly woman continued, seeing Olivia wince as the consultant asked the receptionist something then jabbed a warning finger in the young man's chest.

No way was this man a sweetie. This was a man used to giving orders, and having them obeyed. A man who took life by the scruff of the neck, but never any prisoners, and as from tomorrow she was his boss.

So what? her mind protested when Seth Hardcastle suddenly caught hold of the young man by the lapels and began propelling him towards the exit. *You're the new clinical director in charge of A and E. The whole point of you moving from Edinburgh to Glasgow was to make a fresh start. You were going to be the new super-confident, in-your-face type, remember?*

Except that perhaps she ought to revise the in-your-face bit, she decided as Seth Hardcastle catapulted the young man out into the street. In fact, perhaps she ought to forget about it completely, she thought with a gulp when the consultant turned and cracked a smile at the enthralled waiting room. A smile she felt all the way down to her toes.

'He's wonderful, isn't he?' Her companion beamed.

He was certainly something, Olivia thought as she watched the consultant disappear back into the examination rooms, and yet he hadn't got the clinical director's post. He should have done. At thirty-six he had two years' more experience in A and E than she did, and yet he'd been passed over. Which meant he was flawed in some way.

Not in the attractiveness stakes, her mind whispered, and she stamped on the thought quickly. Lack of commitment? Not judging by the way he'd come to the receptionist's aid. Too abrasive? She shivered, though the waiting room was warm. She certainly wouldn't want him looming over her the way he'd loomed over the young punk.

'Looks like we've got more trouble,' the elderly woman beside her sighed.

Olivia's head snapped round. The waiting room was silent, or as silent as two lustily crying babies and several extremely active children could make it. 'I don't see—'

'Madge is going to make an announcement. That always means trouble.'

Her companion was right. The receptionist was tapping on her desk for attention, and then she cleared her throat.

'I'm sorry, ladies and gentlemen, but there's been a multiple car crash on the A82 south of Loch Lomond. The casualties are on their way to us now so I'm afraid our reviewed waiting time looks likely to be three hours.'

A collective groan of resignation went up from the waiting room, and Olivia bit her lip. Casualties. That could mean anything from two to twenty-two people, and in an emergency A and E needed every qualified member of staff it could get.

She glanced down at her baggy tracksuit bottoms and sweatshirt emblazoned with the words MAKE MY DAY. She was hardly dressed for the occasion but it couldn't be helped. With a sigh she pulled a scrunchie from her handbag, dragged her shoulder-length brown curls back into a ponytail and stood up.

'Leaving, dear?' the woman beside her said.

'In a manner of speaking,' Olivia replied ruefully, and made her way to the reception desk to introduce herself to the receptionist.

'ETA for the casualties ten minutes, Seth,' Sister Babs Grant declared, putting down the phone and reaching for her notepad. 'One severe chest and head injuries, one nasty leg wound, a woman who's fractured both her femurs and a seven-year-old with extensive burns.'

'Burns?' The consultant frowned, and the sister nodded.

'The car he was travelling in caught fire after the pile-up. I've paged Tony, alerted Intensive Care and Theatre's on standby.'

Jerry Swanson grinned. 'Poor Tony. He's only just gone off duty after a sixty-hour shift.'

'Hard work's good for the soul,' Seth observed. 'Especially for the souls of junior doctors. Keeps them off the street and out of the pubs.'

'I bet you didn't think that when you were a junior doctor.' The specialist registrar laughed, and Seth's lips curved.

'Still don't if I'm honest. And speaking of honesty,' he continued as Babs hurried away, 'I don't care what you say. I give this Olivia Mackenzie three months and she'll walk.'

The specialist registrar groaned. 'Seth, you've been gnawing at this particular bone ever since we heard she'd got the job. Dr Mackenzie starts work here tomorrow. Live with it.'

'How?' Seth protested as he strode down the examination room and Jerry followed him. 'It should have been obvious to anyone that A and E's no place for a woman. It's like a battlefield in here some nights and it's tough enough watching our own backs without having to look after a woman as well.'

'Our nurses seem to manage.'

'Only because they know which patients are the trouble-makers and which are the druggies,' Seth argued back. 'This woman will know damn all.'

'Perhaps Admin don't plan on her actually working in the department,' Jerry observed. 'Perhaps they feel we're more in need of a co-ordinator rather than a hands-on consultant.'

'Oh, terrific. That's all we need—another pen-pusher. Three months, Jerry. I'll give her three months, and she'll throw in the towel.'

'She's bought a house in Edmonton Road. Doesn't sound to me like she intends throwing in any towel.'

A frown creased Seth's forehead. 'And we know this how?'

'Charlie in Dietetics happened to see her when she came for her interview. They got talking, and he happened to mention how hard it was to find rented accommodation in Glasgow. She said it wasn't a problem as she'd bought one of those old houses in Edmonton Road.'

'And did Charlie *happen* to find out anything else?' Seth asked caustically.

'Just that she's thirty-four, divorced and seemed nice.'

'Nice?' Seth repeated with exasperation. 'We don't want *nice,* Jerry. We want a tough, committed, hands-on boss, not some wimp who'll run screaming from A and E when a druggy throws up on her, or a roll-over merchant who'll accept all of Admin's crackpot ideas without a murmur.'

Jerry sighed as he erased the name of the last patient he'd seen from the whiteboard. 'Seth, I hate to say this, but this antagonism you seem to feel towards Dr Mackenzie...' He shot his boss a swift, sidelong look. 'It's not simply a bad case of sour grapes, is it?'

Seth opened his mouth, then closed it again. Jerry was right. Dammit, he'd worked in the A and E department of the Belfield Infirmary for the past twelve years. He was good at his job, and to be passed over for a thirty-four-year-old outsider who knew damn all about the department...

'OK, so maybe I *do* think it should have been an inside appointment,' he conceded, suddenly realising that his specialist registrar was waiting for a reply. 'The department has two consult-ants, me and Watson Forrester—'

'Watson still works here?' Jerry eyebrows rose. 'That's going to come as a big surprise to everybody.'

A slight tinge of colour darkened Seth's cheeks. 'OK, so maybe he's not been pulling his weight lately—'

'Seth, he's never here. If he's not off to some conference, he's away at a seminar. He wants out of A and E. You know it, and so do I.'

Seth did, but it didn't make him feel any bet-ter. In fact, it made him feel worse. He gazed round the examination room, at the peeling paint, the tattered cubicle curtains, and bit his lip. 'Jerry, do you ever feel like you're stuck in a rut?'

'Can't say I do. I get the blues occasionally—everybody does—but there's far too much va-riety in A and E for me ever to get bored.'

Once Seth would have agreed with him, but just lately he'd had the worrying feeling that their patients were beginning to merge, to blend, into faceless, nameless anonymity. 'I think I'm getting too old for this job.'

'Seth, you're thirty-six,' Jerry protested. 'You don't get burn-out in A and E until you're fifty.'

'Maybe I should sign up as a doctor on one of those luxury cruise liners,' Seth continued as though his specialist registrar hadn't spoken. 'The ones that sail the Mediterranean or the Caribbean.'

'Dispensing sea-sickness pills and fighting off the advances of the blue-rinse brigade?' Jerry grinned. 'I'd give you a month, and you'd be bored out of your skull.'

'Médicins sans Frontiéres, then,' Seth murmured. 'They're always looking for new doctors.'

Jerry started to laugh, then stopped when he saw his boss was in earnest. 'Okay, let's forget all this crap about Dr Mackenzie, cruise ships, and Médicins sans Frontiéres. What's wrong, Seth—and I mean really wrong?'

The consultant picked up the whiteboard eraser from the table, stared at it for a second, then tossed it down again. 'I don't know—and that's the honest truth. All I do know is nothing seems fun any more. Not my job, not dating, not even sex.' He frowned. 'Especially not sex.'

'I don't see how changing your job is going to make your sex life any better,' Jerry pointed out. 'Look, who are you dating at the moment?'

Seth looked over his shoulder, then lowered his voice. 'Nobody. I haven't been out on a date since June.'

'You haven't had sex for three *months?* Seth—'

'I'm losing it, aren't I?' the consultant exclaimed. 'If I can't even be bothered to have sex any more, I'm definitely losing it.'

Jerry stared thoughtfully at him. 'No, you're not. I think you're just beginning to realise there's more to life than work and a string of casual relationships. I think what you need is to settle down with just one woman.'

'Are you *crazy?*' Seth spluttered. 'The minute a bloke settles down, he's brain dead.'

'Hey, I take great exception to that,' Jerry exclaimed. 'Carol and I have been married for a year, and I'm certainly not brain dead.'

'Not yet, but you soon will be,' Seth said darkly. 'In a couple of years' time your idea of a sparkling evening's entertainment will be sitting in front of the television, poring over some DIY magazines. And when the kids start arriving…' He shuddered. 'I'll ask how they are— just to be polite—and you'll whip out their latest photographs and start telling me all about little Isolde's first tooth and Tristram's first step.'

'That isn't being brain dead,' Jerry said uncertainly. 'It's…it's being proud of your family, loving them, being committed to them.'

It also meant waving goodbye to any exciting foreign holidays because little Isolde didn't like travelling, Seth thought glumly. Goodbye to any visits to a restaurant or to the movies because little Tristram got upset if he was left with a babysitter. And it wasn't just the kids who made you brain dead. It was living with the same woman for the rest of your life, having to see the same face over the breakfast table every morning.

'Seth, listen—'

The consultant couldn't have, even if he'd wanted to. The examination-room doors clattered open and the paramedics who'd attended the multiple car crash appeared, each clamouring for attention.

'Twenty-six-year-old male, Doc. Open leg wound, Glascow coma scale 3-3-4. Blood loss extensive, definite class 11 shock. His saturation levels are falling and he's hardly moving any air.'

'My bloke's in really bad shape, too, Doc,' another paramedic declared. 'Chest and head injuries. GCS 2-2-4. We've tubed him and set up an IV line, but his BP's been falling steadily since we lifted him.'

'Tony—where's Tony?' Seth demanded, and to his relief the junior doctor appeared. He looked as though he'd been dragged out of bed, but at least he was there.

'Seth, the child with the burns needs attention, and fast,' Babs declared, casting her professional eye quickly over the trolleys. 'He's cyanotic for sure.'

The child was. Even from where he was standing Seth could see the characteristic blue tinge of the boy's face which indicated his blood wasn't receiving enough oxygen.

'Jerry, you take the bloke with the head and chest injuries, I'll take the child. Tony, the guy with the open leg wound is yours. Tube him, but keep a careful watch for any signs of a tension pneumothorax or major rupture of his diaphragm.'

'Right,' the junior doctor replied, looking anything but happy.

'What about my patient, Doc?' one of the paramedics protested. 'Diane Lennox, late thirties. She's fractured both her femurs, and I think she could be bleeding internally.'

Seth stared indecisively at the badly burnt child, then across at the female casualty, and exploded. 'This is *ridiculous!* We need another pair of qualified hands. We need another doctor—*any* kind of doctor!'

'Will I do?'

Seth spun round to see a tall, slender woman wearing a pair of baggy tracksuit bottoms and a sweatshirt emblazoned with the words MAKE MY DAY, gazing back at him, and shot a fulminating glance at Madge from Reception who was hovering beside her. 'Madge, could you escort this lady through to the relatives' waiting room? She shouldn't be—'

'Seth, she's not a relative,' the receptionist interrupted. 'She's a bona fide doctor. I've seen her ID, and Admin have verified it. She starts work tomorrow, and she's actually—'

'Boss, I've got the tube in, but this bloke's trachea has definitely shifted to the left,' Tony Melville exclaimed, panic plain in his voice.

'Then he obviously needs a needle thoracotomy,' Seth retorted, more caustically than he'd intended, and the junior doctor flushed.

'I know, but I've never done one before, and...'

Impatiently Seth snapped on a pair of surgical gloves, strode across the examination room and deftly thrust a needle into the patient's chest.

'I'll insert a thoracotomy tube for you in a minute,' he declared when a satisfying hiss of air came from the patient's lungs, 'but in the meantime start him on a two-litre infusion of Ringer's lactate and then get a sterile pad over his leg and apply pressure to stop that bleeding.'

The junior doctor nodded, and Seth swung round to discover that Madge had disappeared and Dr Sweatshirt had not only donned the spare white coat they kept hanging on the back of the examination room door but she'd also slipped an IV line into the badly burnt child's arm and was in the process of inserting a catheter into his bladder.

'What the hell do you think you're doing?' he exclaimed, shooting back across the examination room and elbowing her roughly aside.

'What it looks like,' Dr Sweatshirt protested. 'The child urgently needs fluids to counteract shock, and surely we need to know how much smoke he might have inhaled?'

She was right, but even if her ID was legit that still didn't mean she knew anything about A and E medicine. She could be a dietician or, even worse, a chiropodist.

'What's your specialisation?' he demanded.

'I majored in surgery, but surgery isn't my specialisation now. Look, I think I can set your mind—'

'Paediatrics, or adult?'

'Adult, and if you'd just let me finish—'

'Seth, my head and chest injuries need Neurology,' Jerry called. 'I'm stabilising him as best I can, but he's definitely got an intracranial haematoma.'

'OK, I'll—'

'Seth, could you *please* come and take a look at Mrs Lennox?' Babs exclaimed. 'Her BP's all over the place.'

'I'll be there in a—'

'This child's urine is very dark,' Dr Sweatshirt observed. 'Looks like possible myoglobinuria to me—iron and protein being released from a damaged muscle into his blood and urine. You really should be taking blood samples.'

'And do I look as though I've got six pairs of hands?' Seth exclaimed with frustration, then swore under his breath when a tide of hot colour washed across Dr Sweatshirt's cheeks.

He shouldn't be taking out his frustration on her. It wasn't right, and it wasn't fair. She hadn't needed to offer to help, especially as she didn't officially start work at the Belfield until tomorrow. 'Look, I'm sor—'

'Seth, I really *do* need you,' Babs protested. 'Fiona and I have got an IV line into Mrs Lennox, and we've checked her ABCs, but we're not doctors.'

Ms Sweatshirt was. She'd been right about the possibility of myoglobinuria, and with a specialisation in surgery she probably knew as much—if not more—about burns patients as he did.

'OK, Dr whatever-your-name-is,' he said brusquely. 'Can you take care of the child while I check out Mrs Lennox?'

Dr Sweatshirt nodded. She didn't meet his gaze but she nodded, and he hurried across the examination room.

'I've paged Orthopaedics,' Babs declared. 'Do you want Fiona to get the technicians down for a scan?'

'Yes, please, and, Babs…' He lowered his voice. 'Would you assist Dr Sweatshirt? Watch what she does, and if you're worried—'

'Seth, I'll assist her with pleasure, but you heard what Madge said. She's a bona fide doctor, and she starts work in the hospital tomorrow, so stop stressing. Ye gods, if ever a woman looked as though she knew what she was doing, she does.'

She did, Seth thought as he glanced across at Dr Sweatshirt. She looked calm, in control and completely professional. She was also quite attractive if a man's taste ran to women with soft brown eyes and riotously curly brown hair pulled back into a lopsided ponytail. His didn't. He preferred big-busted blondes with pizzazz, not skinny, wholesome-looking women who looked as though they could have got a part in a remake of *Anne of Green Gables,* but that didn't excuse the fact that he'd been quite unforgivably rude to her.

He sighed as he inserted a catheter into Mrs Lennox's bladder, then checked her femoral pulses. Time for an apology. Time for a quick blast of the old Hardcastle charm.

He cleared his throat pointedly, and saw Dr Sweatshirt's head come up.

'I owe you an apology, don't I?' he said. 'I've been quite appallingly rude to you when you didn't need to volunteer to help, so if you want to lob an IV bag in my direction I promise I won't duck.'

She looked momentarily startled, but when he threw her one of his guaranteed gotta-love-me Hardcastle grins he was the one who blinked when an answering smile slowly curved her lips. Hey, but that smile was quite something. It lit up her face, completely transforming her. Maybe she could be his type after all. Not permanently, of course, because he didn't do permanence, but maybe for dinner tonight, a few dates...

'I've just realised I don't even know your name,' he said, upping his smile a notch. 'I'm Seth Hardcastle, A and E consultant, and you are—'

'OK, which of you jokers called for a brain expert?'

Seth turned to see the consultant from Neurology standing in the doorway, and laughed. 'Jerry did, but I wouldn't say no to a quick brain transplant.'

'I don't do freebies, Seth.' The consultant grinned, but as he walked towards Jerry it wasn't Seth who sighed but Olivia.

She needed a quick brain transplant too or, perhaps more accurately, a quick course in self-assertiveness. She should have told Seth Hardcastle who she was. She should have said, Look, sunshine, I'm your boss, but the trouble was she'd never been the 'Look, sunshine' type. She'd always favoured the softly-softly approach both in her personal and her professional

life, coaxing by persuasion rather than by con-
frontation, and it had worked. Well, it had
worked in her professional life at any rate.

'Liv, Phil was a jerk, and you divorced him,'
Deborah had said. 'Get over it, move on.' And
she would. Eventually. But six months wasn't
nearly long enough to forget that the man who
had promised to love and cherish her had been
bedding his secretary on a depressingly regular
basis throughout their short married life.

'Are you all right?'

Babs was gazing at her curiously, and Olivia
forced a smile.

'I'm fine. It's just... Is the department always
this chaotic?'

The sister chuckled. 'You should see us on a
Saturday night. I don't know how we'd manage
without Seth and Jerry.'

Jerry Swanson. The department's specialist
registrar. Thirty-two and married to one of the
nurses in Women's Surgical, according to his
file. She could handle him, but Seth
Hardcastle...

The trouble was he looked even more im-
pressive up close than he'd done in the waiting
room. He shouldn't have done. His blue eyes
were bloodshot, his chin was dark with stubble
and his black hair was falling carelessly over his

forehead. He looked as though he hadn't slept for days. He also looked as sexy as hell, and it wasn't a reassuring combination.

'I know Seth can be a bit abrasive,' the sister continued, clearly misinterpreting her silence, 'but he's one of the best consultants I've ever worked with.'

And if I don't toughen up, he's going to walk right over me, Olivia thought as she heard Seth snap at something Tony Melville had said.

'Oh, hallelujah,' Babs exclaimed with relief. 'Here come the crispy squad.'

The crispy squad. The irreverent name most A and E units gave to the burns unit. The crispy squad would take care of the little boy, Neurology was attending to the chest and head case, and Seth and Jerry could look after Mrs Lennox and the man with the open leg wound. She wasn't needed any more. She could simply slip away, and she fully intended doing just that when she suddenly heard Seth say her name.

'I'm afraid Seth's on his high horse about our new clinical director,' Babs said ruefully as a slight crease furrowed Olivia's forehead. 'He's not very happy at her appointment.'

Not very happy was the understatement of the year, Olivia thought as she heard Jerry declare, 'Look, all I said was I can't see Admin appointing somebody with no A and E experience,' and Seth flashing back, 'Well, if she's not a pen-pusher, I bet her so-called experience consists of performing unnecessary cosmetic operations on women with more money than sense.'

A spurt of anger flared inside Olivia as she stared at the consultant's irate face, a spurt she hadn't felt since she'd found out about Phil's extra-marital affair. Just who the hell did Seth Hardcastle think he was? Well, she might not be able to tell him who he was, but she sure as shooting could tell him *what* he was.

She strode across the examination room, her brown eyes flashing, and arrived in time to hear Seth declare, 'Just don't come complaining to me when you discover she's as much use as a plastic bag in a thunderstorm. This woman—'

'This woman feels she ought to introduce herself before you say anything else,' Olivia interrupted, her voice ice-cold. 'I'm Olivia Mackenzie, your new pen-pushing clinical director.'

Jerry let out an anguished groan, but Seth didn't look one bit discomfited. Instead, he met her gaze squarely.

'I suppose you're expecting an apology?'

'Well, your manners could certainly do with some work—'

'We don't have time for manners in A and E, Dr Mackenzie, not when our patients are often bleeding like stuck pigs.'

'No, but you seem to have plenty of time to bad-mouth a colleague behind her back,' she snapped. 'For your information, I worked for ten years in the A and E department of the Edinburgh General, and even if I hadn't I would have expected you to extend me the courtesy of at least meeting me before you tore my character to shreds!'

A wash of bright colour flooded across Seth's cheeks, and Olivia only just restrained herself from punching the air in triumph. She'd taken the wind right out of his sails, and it hadn't been hard. In fact, it had been easy. She could be the in-your-face type after all, and it felt wonderful.

'I...um... Our shift finishes in half an hour, Dr Mackenzie,' Jerry Swanson said, far too brightly. 'Would you like to stick around, join us for coffee in the staffroom?'

Seth didn't second the suggestion. From his rigid expression she reckoned he was probably too busy wishing her dead.

'I'm afraid I can't,' she said, summoning up her most gracious smile for the specialist registrar. 'I told George I wouldn't be long, and he must be wondering where I am.'

And with a nod to Babs and Tony Melville, she turned on her heel and walked out of the examination room, knowing Seth's eyes were following her the whole way.

'Arrogant, rude, obnoxious man,' she muttered to herself as she drove home. 'Somebody should have chopped him down to size years ago, and I don't take back a word of what I said. I *don't.*'

George clearly agreed with her when she told him all about it. At least, he followed her into the kitchen, keeping his eyes fixed firmly on her, which sort of suggested he agreed.

'It's not a bad department, George,' she told him as she slid a chill-cook curry into the microwave. 'Their treat and street times are far too long, and the waiting room is a disgrace, but at least they all seem to know what they're doing. Even Seth Hardcastle.'

Actually, especially Seth Hardcastle, she thought, pausing as she reached for two bowls. He was obviously a first-rate consultant. A first-rate and now extremely angry consultant. Maybe she shouldn't have been quite so in-your-face. Maybe she ought to have approached the situation differently. Maybe….

Oh, for crying out loud. Who's the new clinical director here—you or him? He had no right

*to be talking about you behind your back, so
stop being a wimp. You were a wimp for two
years with Phil, and look where that got you.*

She glanced down at George. 'Do you think
I went too far—said too much?'

He stared back at her uncomprehendingly for
a second, then put his shaggy head down on his
paws, and she sighed.

That was the trouble with dogs. No verbal
reassurances, no bracing words of encourage-
ment when you most needed them. They might
be more loving and loyal than the average husband, but great conversationalists they weren't.

Unlike her sister, she thought when the phone
rang and she went out into the hall to answer it.

'I just thought I'd phone to wish you the best
of luck for tomorrow,' Deborah exclaimed,
bright and cheerful as always.

Her sister thought she needed luck? Maybe
after meeting Seth Hardcastle she did. No, she
didn't. She was the new super-confident, in-
your-face Olivia Mackenzie. 'Deb—'

'Harry says he still can't understand why you
had to move from Edinburgh to Glasgow. He
says there's lots of clinical directors' posts in
Edinburgh in nice hospitals in nice areas.'

Her brother-in-law the snob. 'Deb—'

'Liv, all I want is for you to be happy. I know Phil dumped you for a twenty-four-year-old blonde with a 36D cup and an eighteen-inch waist, but that doesn't mean you should give up on men. You're bright and kind, and lots of men prefer brains to looks.'

Olivia met George's gaze. She'd been wrong. Talking to a dog was sometimes infinitely preferable to talking to a human being.

'Deb, I have to go—my dinner's ready,' she lied.

'OK, but promise me you'll keep your eyes open for any dishy-looking men. *Ciao,* Liv.'

The phone went dead before Olivia could tell her sister that nobody said 'Ciao' or 'dishy' any more, and that the last thing she wanted was a man, dishy or otherwise.

You won't even have to look, a little voice at the back of her mind reminded her as her microwave pinged. As from tomorrow you'll have the most incredibly dishy-looking man working right under your nose.

'Terrific,' she said without enthusiasm, and George wagged his tail in agreement.

CHAPTER TWO

'THAT has to be the most ridiculous suggestion I've ever heard!' Seth exclaimed, and Olivia gritted her teeth until they hurt.

A week. She'd been at the Belfield Infirmary for exactly one week, and Seth Hardcastle had disagreed with every plan she'd put forward to improve the running of the department. Good grief, he'd even argued against redecorating the waiting room when it must have been obvious to anyone that the place was a dump.

'It is *not* a ridiculous suggestion,' she said with difficulty. 'The health department has conducted a survey—'

'Oh, well, if they've conducted a *survey.*'

'And sixty-five per cent of the general public object to their names being written up on a whiteboard,' she continued, deliberately ignoring his sarcasm. 'They feel it's an invasion of their privacy.'

Seth leant back in his seat and folded his arms across his chest. 'An invasion of their privacy. Right. And if we remove the whiteboard, just how—precisely—are we supposed to identify patients?'

'By communicating with each other, of course,' she snapped, and saw his lip curl.

'So, on a busy Saturday night, when we're full to capacity, and somebody's bleeding to death on one trolley and somebody's having a coronary on another, we're supposed to make time for these illuminating conversations, are we?'

Olivia dug her clenched fingers deep into the pockets of her white coat, but it didn't help. Why did their morning meetings have to always end like this in acrimony and disagreement? The rest of the A and E department had made her feel welcome, but Seth… He never stopped arguing, and it wasn't just the arguing which was getting her down. It was his unerring ability to make her feel small and stupid. A feeling which wasn't helped this morning by her sneaking suspicion that he was right about the whiteboard, and the health board's directive *was* crazy.

'Whether you approve of the whiteboard coming down or not, it is coming down,' she said tightly. 'And speaking of coming down,' she continued as he opened his mouth, clearly intending to argue. 'Watson Forrester.'

He stirred uncomfortably in his seat. 'What about Watson?'

She picked up one of the folders on her desk and extracted a sheet of paper from it. 'According to this, he's been to two seminars, three conferences and four courses this year.'

A faint flush of colour seeped across Seth's cheeks. 'Watson likes to keep abreast of the latest A and E developments.'

'By going to conferences on food nutrition?' He winced and her battered self-esteem sent up a silent *Yeah!* of triumph. 'I want his resignation, Seth,' she said quickly, before he had time to come up with one of his crushing put-downs. 'He's in London for another couple of days on this food nutrition course, then he's off on his annual leave, but when he comes back I want his resignation.'

Seth looked as though he'd like to argue, but he also looked as though he knew when he was beaten. Being beaten, however, didn't stop him from muttering, 'You'll be wanting Jerry's resignation next.' She closed the folder with a snap.

'Certainly not. He's an excellent specialist registrar. In fact, the whole team works very well together, including young Tony Melville.'

'You think so?'

Something about his tone brought a slight crease to her forehead. 'You don't?' He didn't reply, and her frown deepened. 'Look, if there's something I should know about Tony, I'd far rather you just told me.'

He opened his mouth, closed it again and shook his head. 'It's nothing—just a gut feeling.'

'A gut feeling you're clearly not prepared to share with me,' she said icily. 'Fine. If that's the way you want to play it.'

'I'm not playing anything,' he protested. 'I just don't think I ought to condemn the guy without concrete facts.'

It was on the tip of her tongue to say that hadn't prevented him from bad-mouthing her, but she didn't. Persuasion, Olivia, she told herself. You've always succeeded in the past with even the stroppiest of consultants by using the gentle art of persuasion, so back off. Back off, and regroup.

She fixed a conciliatory smile to her lips. 'I think I've covered everything I want to discuss this morning. Is there anything you'd like to talk to me about?'

'No.'

Not an 'I don't think so' or an 'I can't think of anything'—just a bald, flat 'No'. Couldn't he even pretend to be civil, attempt to meet her halfway? Apparently not, judging by the rigid set of his jaw. Well, irrespective of how he felt, they couldn't permanently be at loggerheads. They had to find some common ground or they would never be able to work together.

'Listen, Seth,' she declared, doing her best to radiate sympathy and understanding, which wasn't easy when what she really felt like doing was hitting him. 'I know this can't be easy for you—having me as your boss. You're bound to feel slightly resentful—'

'I don't feel even remotely resentful,' he interrupted. 'I just don't think a woman should be in charge of A and E.'

Her jaw dropped. Was he kidding? He didn't look as though he was, and her sympathy and understanding disappeared in an instant.

'Now, listen here,' she exclaimed, her brown eyes stormy. 'It may have escaped your attention—it clearly *has* escaped your attention—but women moved out of the kitchen years ago. There are women politicians, women judges, women consultants—'

'I'm quite aware of that,' he exclaimed, annoyance plain in his voice, 'and I have no objection to female consultants in principle. The

head of Ophthalmics is a woman. The head of
Geriatrics is a woman—'

'You just don't want one in your own back
yard,' she finished for him furiously. 'Well, I'm
sorry, but I'm here for the duration, and you and
your fragile male ego are just going to have to
get used to it!'

Yikes, but where had that come from? she
wondered, seeing anger darken his blue eyes.
She'd never been the confrontational type.
Deborah was always telling her she was too
darned soft for her own good, but this man...
He constantly seemed to bring out the worst in
her.

Which didn't mean she was going to apologise.

Dammit, why should she? If he was a chau-
vinist—and she'd never in a million years have
pegged him as one—then he was going to have
to learn she wasn't a pushover.

Or at least not a complete one, she thought,
forcing herself not to flinch back in her seat
when he got to his feet and his broad shoulders
blocked out the sunlight from her window.

'Seth, listen—'

'My shift starts in half an hour, and I'd like
a coffee before I go on duty, so if there's nothing else, Dr Mackenzie...?'

He couldn't even call her Olivia. Everybody else did. Jerry, Tony, Babs, Fiona. Only Seth seemed unable—or unwilling—to force her name through his teeth.

'Seth—'

'I really would like that coffee.'

It was hopeless, she thought as she gazed up into his implacable face. Completely and utterly hopeless.

'I'll see you later, then,' she said, and without a word, or even so much as a nod, he was gone.

Stupid, pompous, arrogant man. What on earth was she going to do with him? If they couldn't establish a decent working relationship she would have to ask for his resignation, and she didn't want his resignation. He was an excellent consultant. Skilled, intuitive, unflappable.

Handsome, too, her mind whispered as she gathered up the folders on her desk and she let out a huff of impatience. OK, so he was handsome, and when he smiled... Not that he'd done any smiling in her direction during the past week, but she'd seen him smile at Babs and Fiona, and it was the kind of smile that did odd things to a woman's stomach.

'Odd things to her brain, too,' she murmured out loud as she put the folders in her filing cabinet and closed the drawer with a bang. 'Face it, Liv. A man like Seth Hardcastle would leave you emotionally scarred for life.'

Yes, but think of the fun while it lasted.

Don't think of the fun, she told herself severely as she walked out of her office and down to the examination room. The only thing you want from Seth Hardcastle is a good working relationship. Nothing more, nothing less.

There didn't seem to be much work going on in A and E when she opened the door. In fact, there didn't seem to be any work going on at all, just Babs and Fiona crouched up against the back wall surrounded by a mass of squashed fruit.

'What on earth's going on?' Olivia asked, only to duck quickly as a pear suddenly came shooting out of cubicle 6 followed by the sound of a male voice calling, 'Cock-a-doodle-doo!'

'Brian Taylor,' Babs replied. 'He came in with a badly cut hand, and Fiona and I had just got a saline drip into him when all hell broke loose.'

'He's one of our regulars, and a chronic alcoholic,' the staff nurse chipped in. 'We reckon he's been on one of his three-day benders.'

'Which doesn't alter the fact that his hand needs stitching,' Olivia said firmly. 'Why haven't you sedated him?'

A watermelon sailed out of the cubicle and landed with a dull thud at Babs's feet.

'Because we'd rather like to finish the day in one piece,' the sister replied. 'So if you have any bright ideas on how we can get close enough to him...'

It was a good point. It was also at times like this that Olivia wished she was a man. Preferably a six-foot-two-inch tall man with broad shoulders and blue eyes, but if she paged Seth he'd never let her forget it.

'Where are Jerry and Tony?' she asked.

'Jerry's in cubicle 1 with a possible duodenal, and Tony's trying to figure out what's wrong with the woman in 3.'

Which meant she was on her own.

Well, brawn wasn't everything, she told herself. In fact, the voice of sweet reason could often be surprisingly effective.

'Mr Taylor?' she called out in her most re-assuring voice. A bunch of bananas came hurtling through the curtains, and he started cock-a-doodling again. 'What's he got in there, Babs?' she hissed. 'The entire contents of a fruit shop?'

The sister grinned. 'We're just hoping he didn't stop off at his local fishmonger's before he came here.'

Olivia fervently hoped so, too. She chewed her lip for a second, then made up her mind. 'I need a syringe loaded with the strongest sedative you've got.'

Babs did as she asked, but when Olivia pocketed the syringe and got down on her hands and knees, the sister eyed her uncertainly. 'Are you sure about this? I could call Seth—'

Over her dead body. 'Of course I'm sure,' Olivia replied, but she didn't feel anything like as confident when she crawled into the cubicle and caught sight of Mr Taylor sitting on top of the trolley.

Dear lord, but he was huge. If he stopped throwing fruit and started throwing his fists, she was going to be in serious trouble.

Think positive, Olivia, she told herself firmly. You might not have physical strength but you have intelligence. And probably about ten seconds in which to use it, she calculated as she stretched up, yanked the saline drip off its hook and then crouched down again fast.

Make that five seconds, she amended with a sinking heart as an ominous rustling sound came from the trolley, which suggested that Mr Taylor was delving into his shopping bag again.

'There's no need to get agitated, Mr Taylor,' she said soothingly. 'I'm here to help you.'

'Get lost!'

'And I love you, too,' she muttered under her breath as she swiftly injected the syringe full of sedative into the drip tube. 'Now, if you could just breathe in deeply for me, I'll—'

She didn't get a chance to finish what she'd been about to say. Tomatoes began raining down on her, splattering her white coat, and she squeezed on the saline bag for all she was worth. It was a quick-acting sedative, but he was a big man and it could be several seconds before it took effect. All she could hope was that it kicked in before he ran out of tomatoes.

'Sleepy time, Mr Taylor,' she crooned. 'Time to go to the land of nod. Time for Mr Sandman to come along and close your eyes.'

'Get lost,' he said again, but this time with slightly less enthusiasm, and she squeezed even harder on the bag.

'Maybe you should consider visiting the Merkland Memorial next time you injure yourself,' she continued. 'Much as we love having your custom...'

Bingo! With a surprising grace for such a big man, Mr Taylor keeled over on the trolley, and she caught his bag of groceries just before it hit the floor.

A smile curved her lips. She'd been right. Brawn wasn't everything. Brains could be just as effective, but it had been a close-run thing.

'OK, Mr Tough Guy,' she murmured, getting awkwardly to her feet. 'Let's see what damage you've done to yourself.'

To her relief his hand wasn't as badly injured as it had looked. He'd certainly sliced his thumb pretty badly, and there were lacerations to his other fingers, but luckily he hadn't hit any vital arteries.

'You must have a charmed life,' she observed as she cleaned his hand, then inserted some stitches. 'Pity I can't say the same about your manners.' A loud snore was her only reply and she chuckled. 'See you around, Mr Taylor—but hopefully not for a very long time.'

Quickly she pulled back the cubicle curtains and blinked as a round of applause greeted her.

'Way to go, boss!' Babs beamed. 'Whoever said women were the weaker species?'

'Not at the Belfield they're not,' Fiona exclaimed, and Jerry grinned.

'You look as though you've had a tussle with a mad axe murderer and lost.'

'Oh, *fun*ny.' Olivia laughed. 'Babs, Mr Taylor's hand will need a dressing. I've given him enough sedative to knock out an elephant but keep your eye on him. He—'

'What the hell's going on?'

Olivia turned to see Seth striding down the examination room towards her, and smiled. 'Crisis over. Mr Taylor—'

'You're bleeding,' Seth declared, concern plain on his face. 'Babs, we'll need a cross-match, X-rays—'

'Seth, these are tomato stains,' Olivia said, beginning to laugh, only to stop when she saw his expression. 'I'm not laughing at you—honestly I'm not. It was sweet of you to be concerned, but Mr Taylor just decided to throw some fruit around, and I was the unlucky recipient of the tomatoes. I've stitched—'

'Babs, have you telephoned the janitor to come and clean up this mess?' he snapped, cutting right across Olivia's explanation.

The sister flushed. 'Not yet, but—'

'Then I suggest you do it now. If a patient slips and falls we'll have a negligence suit slapped on us before you can say diddly squat and I don't think Admin will consider *that* a laughing matter, do you?'

'And I don't think there was any need for you to chew poor Babs's head off,' Olivia protested as the sister hurried towards the phone and Fiona escaped into Mr Taylor's cubicle. 'It's been pretty hairy in here for the past quarter of an hour, and—' He'd walked away from her. He'd just upped and walked away, and she turned to Jerry furiously. 'Of all the rude, arrogant… What is *wrong* with that guy?'

'I think he was worried about you,' the specialist registrar replied, and Olivia rolled her eyes heavenwards.

'*Worried?* Seth Hardcastle wouldn't care if I was strung up by a mob of rioting yobs.'

'Of course he would. Look, he's not normally like this,' Jerry continued as Olivia shook her head. 'All right, so he can be a bit abrasive at times if he thinks a patient's trying to con him, or if Admin's giving him the runaround, but—'

'So you're saying it's me—my fault?' Olivia exclaimed, pulling off her stained white coat and throwing it into the laundry basket with rather more force than was strictly necessary. 'Jerry, he's *impossible*. If I said white, he'd say black, just to be difficult.'

The specialist registrar looked uncomfortable. 'I know he has some pretty strong views—'

'*Some?*' Olivia spluttered. She opened her mouth to give Jerry chapter and verse of all the things Seth had said and done over the past week, then snapped her jaw shut. Gossiping with a member of staff about another member of staff was a definite no-no. Asking for information, however, wasn't. 'Jerry, why didn't he get the clinical director's job? He's got the experience, the ability, so why didn't he get the job?'

Jerry sighed. 'Seth's always been a bit of a maverick, and I guess Admin's not keen on guys doing their own thing.'

Independence wasn't a bad thing, Olivia thought as she stared down the examination room to where Seth was deep in conversation with one of the nurses. She just wished his particular brand of independence wasn't always constantly directed at her.

'Well, I can't change my sex,' she said belligerently, 'so he's just going to have to live with it.'

Jerry looked startled. 'Can't change your…? Why would you—?'

'Oh, lord, what's wrong *now?*' Olivia ex-claimed as Tony strode angrily out of cubicle 3, followed by an equally irate-looking man.

'Looks like young Tony's in trouble,' Jerry observed.

'Looks like young Tony needs help,' Olivia said, and together they hurried towards him.

'Dr Mackenzie, perhaps you can convince Mr Carter that I'm a bona fide, fully qualified medic,' Tony said the moment he saw her. 'He seems to feel—'

'Is either of you somebody in authority?' Mr Carter demanded, glancing from Jerry to Olivia then back again.

'I'm the clinical director in charge of this de-partment,' Olivia replied. 'What can I do for you?'

'*You're* in charge of the department?'

The man's surprise was palpable, and Olivia gritted her teeth for the third time that morning. Where were all these New Age men she kept reading about? Her tally for today—and it wasn't even eleven o'clock yet—was two male chauvinists and a drunk who thought women should be used as target practice.

'Yes, I'm in charge of the department,' she said as evenly as she could. 'What seems to be the trouble?'

'There *is* no trouble,' Tony insisted. 'I'm just trying to convince Mr Carter that his wife has a bad cold—'

'My wife does *not* have a cold,' Mr Carter interrupted. 'My wife is ill—very ill—and I want a second opinion.'

Out of the corner of her eye Olivia could see that Seth was no longer talking to the nurse but staring intently at the whiteboard. He didn't fool her for a second. He was eavesdropping, listening to find out how she was going to handle the situation. Well, let him listen. She didn't need his help. If she could deal with a fruit-throwing alcoholic, she could deal with an irate husband.

She beckoned to Babs. 'Sister, could you take Mr Carter—?'

'I'm not going anywhere,' the man exclaimed, his eyes angry, his colour high. 'I'm staying right here until you find out what's wrong with my wife.'

He would, too, unless she found some way to placate him, and Olivia summoned up one of her best trust-me-I'm-a-doctor smiles. 'I'm afraid it's against hospital policy for us to examine a patient while a relative is present.'

'He didn't say that,' Mr Carter protested, gesturing at Tony. 'In fact, he—'

'It's written into my contract,' Olivia declared, and saw Seth's lips twitch. OK, so it was a feeble excuse but if Tony's diagnosis was wrong, the last thing she wanted was Mr Carter present when she discovered it. 'I'll be as fast as I can, Mr Carter,' she continued, upping her smile a notch. 'And the second I've made my diagnosis you'll be the first to know.'

That Mr Carter didn't want to go was plain, but Olivia kept on smiling, kept on radiating confidence, and eventually he reluctantly followed Babs out of the examination room.

'OK, what have we got?' Olivia said, turning to Tony.

'Mrs Carter's shivering, she's slightly feverish and she has a headache. She has all the classic symptoms of a cold.'

She also had all the classic symptoms of something else, Olivia realised when she'd finished examining the woman.

'*Malaria?*' the junior doctor gasped. 'You think she has *malaria?*'

'Didn't you notice how brown she was?' Olivia said. 'We might have had a good summer, but there's no way she could have got that suntan in Glasgow. My guess is she's been to Africa or Asia, and that's where she contracted the disease.'

The junior doctor stared unhappily at her. 'I feel like an idiot.'

'Don't,' Olivia protested. 'Good grief, it's not as though malaria's so rampant in Glasgow that even our janitor would have recognised it. And we don't even know for certain yet that she *has* malaria,' she continued when Tony didn't cheer up, 'so why don't you take some blood samples and get them checked by the lab?'

With a nod and a worried frown Tony hurried back into the cubicle, and as Olivia pulled off her examination gloves Jerry stared at her thoughtfully.

'That was a very kind thing to do. A lot of consultants would have nailed him to the wall for a mistake like that.'

'I've seen a couple of cases of malaria before,' Olivia replied dismissively. 'He hasn't.'

'It was still a kind thing to do,' Jerry insisted, and Olivia's eyes flicked across the examination room to where Seth was still hovering by the whiteboard.

'Believe it or not, I'm actually quite a nice person. And now I'd better find out how Mr Taylor's doing,' she continued, 'before some people accuse me of not pulling my weight.'

She'd gone before Jerry could reply and the specialist registrar shook his head as Seth walked across to him. 'You asked for that.'

'What makes you think she meant me?' Seth demanded.

Jerry gave him a hard stare. 'Seth, I'd have to be blind and deaf not to see you're never off her back. She's smart, on the ball and more than pulls her weight in the department, so what's your problem?'

Seth opened his mouth, clearly thought the better of what he'd been about to say and muttered grimly, 'She said I was sweet. I am *not* sweet.'

Jerry laughed. 'Yes, you are. You're nothing but a big pussy cat at heart, so stop riling her.'

'*Me* rile her?' Seth choked. 'Listen, Jerry—'

'I like her.'

'Fine. Feel free to have a mad, passionate affair with her, and when Carol slices off your reproductive organs with a scalpel, don't say I didn't warn you.'

'Carol knows I wouldn't cheat on her, and I won't.' The specialist registrar glanced down the examination room to where Olivia was talking to Fiona. 'She is pretty, though, isn't she?'

She was, Seth thought as he followed the direction of the specialist registrar's gaze. Not beautiful—her nose was too small and her chin was too pointed for beauty—but she was pretty in a gentle, homespun sort of way, and when she smiled... 'She's OK.'

'You thought she was a lot better than OK when you first saw her.'

He had, but that had been before he'd discovered who she was. 'She's too skinny.'

Jerry tilted his head and surveyed Olivia critically. 'Slender. Not skinny—slender. And she's got great legs.'

She had. Long legs. Endless legs. The kind of legs a man could fantasise about. The kind of legs guaranteed to give a man wet dreams.

'I've never been a leg man myself,' Seth lied. 'And even if I was,' he added quickly as Jerry's eyebrows rose, 'she's already in a relationship.'

'Says who?'

'She did last week. Some guy called George.'

'Oh. Right.' Jerry's eyes drifted down the examination room again. 'Pity.'

'I doubt if Carol would think so,' Seth said testily, and Jerry grinned.

'I'm not thinking of me, you dummy. I was thinking of you.'

'Hey, who are you calling a dummy?' Seth protested, but the specialist registrar was already hurrying away in answer to Babs's call.

He wasn't a dummy. He just had a healthy sense of self-preservation. OK, so Olivia had a pair of incredible legs and nice eyes, but dating your boss was asking for trouble. Dating your boss on a strictly let's-have-fun-for-a-few-dates-and-then-it's-over basis was career suicide.

Not that she'd ever go out with him, he thought ruefully as he watched all laughter disappear from her face when she noticed him staring at her. She thought he was a jerk, and he was. All the crap he'd given her about how it ought to have been a man appointed clinical director. He didn't give a damn that she was a woman. What really bugged him was she'd got the job, and he hadn't.

'Childish,' he muttered out loud. 'No, not you, Tony,' he added quickly, seeing the startled look on the junior doctor's face as he emerged from Mrs Carter's cubicle clutching a blood sample. 'Me.'

And he *was* being childish, he thought as the junior doctor scurried away.

Jerry was right. Olivia more than pulled her weight in the department, and she was spunky, too. Lord, just thinking about her tackling Brian Taylor was enough to make him shudder. The man was unpredictable enough when he was sober, but when he was drunk...

And she'd been terrific with young Tony. Any other consultant would have torn the junior doctor to shreds. He probably would have done so himself, and yet Olivia had taken the softly-softly approach, ensuring the young man's confidence wasn't shattered.

He'd have to apologise to her, but apologising would mean telling her why he'd behaved as he had, and she'd think he was a jerk, and he didn't want her thinking he was a jerk.

'Something wrong?' Babs asked curiously, seeing him frown as she passed, and he shook his head.

'Nothing I can't fix,' he replied lightly, but who was he kidding? It was going to take a lot more than one of his smiles to smooth down Olivia's ruffled feathers. But what?

Nothing occurred to him as he treated the elderly woman with the worst case of haemorrhoids he'd ever seen. No solution presented itself when he patched up the victim of a horrific car crash, and because he couldn't think of anything his temper grew shorter and shorter and it was a relief to everyone when their shift finally ended.

'Boy, but Seth's been a little ray of sunshine today, hasn't he?' Jerry observed when Olivia helped him to gather up the notes on the patients they'd seen that day.

'What do you mean, "today"?' she replied. The specialist registrar chuckled, but his laughter faded as he saw Seth striding towards them with a look of grim determination plain on his face.

'Want me to stick around, act as a referee?' he murmured. 'Or, then again, perhaps not,' he added, his smile returning as Olivia shot him a look that spoke volumes. 'OK, I'm out of here.'

Lucky you, Olivia thought with a deep sigh, but if Seth thought he was going to bend her ear for the next half-hour he was very much mistaken.

'Five minutes,' she said as soon as he came to a halt in front of her. 'You've got exactly five minutes, and then I'm going home.'

'Five minutes is all I need,' he replied, shouldering open the examination-room door then standing back so she could walk out into the corridor ahead of him.

It had better be, she thought grimly.

'OK, what's so important that it won't wait until tomorrow?' she demanded, once they were both standing outside in the corridor.

'I just wanted to say how much I admired the way you dealt with Tony this morning—not ripping into him when the lab confirmed Mrs Carter's malaria.'

Praise from Seth Hardcastle? That had to be a first, and he also looked uncomfortable. He never looked uncomfortable. He was up to something.

'I'm glad you approve,' she said. 'Now, if there's nothing else—'

'I also think you were right when you said we needed to talk. We do need to talk, Olivia.'

He'd called her by her first name. He'd praised her, and he'd called her by her first name. He was *definitely* up to something.

'What kind of talking?' she said warily.

'I think we need to talk about us.'

Us? As in him and her? His blue eyes were fixed on her, dark, and liquid and fathomless, and she swallowed—hard. Surely he wasn't going to hit on her? He must know she'd knock him back. She was his boss, and relationships between staff members never worked, and she didn't want to get involved with him anyway, and...

'Seth—'

'We always seem to be arguing, and I don't want us to argue.'

Neither did she but, oh, lord, now he was smiling at her. That heart-stopping smile she hadn't seen since last week. The smile which did odd things to her stomach and made her toes curl.

She took a steadying breath. 'I don't want to argue with you either, but—'

'So I think there's only one thing we can do.'

Oh, cripes, he *was* going to hit on her, and it wouldn't work, she knew it wouldn't. OK, so he was jaw-droppingly attractive but she didn't do casual relationships, and he didn't do permanence, and though a fling with him might be fun—hell, of course it would be fun—the repercussions didn't bear thinking about.

'What...?' Her voice had come out way too high, and she cleared her throat and started again. 'What—exactly—did you have in mind?'

'A truce.'

A truce. Not 'Why don't we have a wild passionate affair?' but a truce. Well, of course she'd known deep down that he wasn't going to suggest an affair. Good grief, they'd only known each other a week, and she wasn't his type, but...

'Sounds good to me,' she said, suddenly realising he was waiting for a reply. 'What sort of a truce did you have in mind?'

He leant back against the corridor wall. 'That you agree I might occasionally be right because of the length of time I've worked here, and I agree *you* might occasionally be right because you're seeing everything with fresh eyes.'

It made sense. It made a lot of sense. A niggling voice at the back of her head pointed out that he could still be up to something, but she decided to meet him halfway.

'Agreed,' she said.

He stuck out his hand. 'Shake on it?'

Try as she may, she couldn't prevent a chuckle springing to her lips. 'Shake on it,' she agreed, and put her hand in his.

It was a mistake. She knew the minute their fingers touched that it was a mistake. Her hand felt so safe in his. Safe, and warm, and protected, and any woman who thought she was safe with Seth Hardcastle needed her head examined. He was breath-taking sex on legs, and trouble and heartache, and she'd had more than enough trouble and heartache to last her a lifetime.

But not enough breath-taking sex, her body whispered. Sex with Phil had been dull and unsatisfying, whereas sex with Seth... No, she wasn't even going to speculate about what sex with Seth would be like, and quickly she eased her fingers free from his, praying her cheeks weren't as red as they felt.

'I have to go. George—'

'Ah, yes. I'd forgotten about George.'

His voice sounded oddly flat, and she wondered if he didn't like dogs. Phil hadn't. He'd pretended to like George, and George had pretended to like him, and then she'd discovered Phil had only been pretending to love her and her marriage had ended.

'I really must go,' she said, backing up a step.

'I must, too,' he replied, not moving at all.

'I'll see you tomorrow, then,' she mumbled, and he nodded, and she walked briskly down the corridor.

I am not going to look back, she told herself. *Looking back is what teenagers do when they're desperate to know whether the boy they're interested in might be interested in them so I'm not going to look back.*

But she did.

Just as she pushed open the door leading to the car park she glanced over her shoulder, and he was still there, still watching her, and his face creased into a smile. A smile that had her smiling back like some dippy, moonstruck, sixteen-year-old. A smile that had her heart doing a happy quickstep. As she stepped out into the open air, she muttered out loud to nobody in particular, 'Oh, damn.'

CHAPTER THREE

'So I'm looking at this two-month-old baby who's covered in greenish-yellow vomit, and my brain's working overtime,' Seth declared as he spooned some coffee into a mug. 'Could it have a strangulated hernia, Crohn's disease, or maybe the child's suffering from inflammatory bowel disease?'

'And what was wrong?' Olivia asked, knowing full well from the twinkle in Seth's blue eyes that the baby hadn't been suffering from any of the conditions he'd mentioned.

'It transpires that forgetful Mum ran out of baby formula, so what does clueless Dad suggest? That banana and kiwi milkshake would make a good alternative. Frankly, I think adoption would be a better alternative for the poor mite, but unfortunately it's not an option.'

Olivia spluttered with laughter. 'What age were these idiots?'

'Eighteen, but as we all know only too well neither age nor social class count when it comes to full-blown idiocy,' Seth replied as he carried his cup of coffee across the staffroom and sat down. 'Jerry, do you remember that kid who suffered third-degree burns after she poked a knitting needle into a wall socket? Turned out she'd done it dozens of times before but her middle-class, middle-aged parents hadn't installed socket plugs because they didn't want to stunt her creativity.'

Jerry nodded as he bit into his sandwich. 'My favourite's still the kid who stuck his grandma's hearing aid up his bum, and when we got it back Grandma lodged a formal complaint because it didn't work any more.'

'You're kidding?' Olivia gasped, and Seth laughed.

'You should know better than that.'

She did, but as she joined in his laughter, all she could think was how wonderful it was to be able to laugh with him. Their truce had been in place now for over a week, and it had made such a difference to be able to talk to him without arguing all the time.

That's not the only thing you find wonderful, her body whispered as Seth leant forward to select a biscuit and his shirt tightened across his chest.

Oh, grow up, she told herself, taking a deep gulp of her coffee and an even bigger lungful of air. *OK, so he's seriously attractive, and the*

*thought of jumping into bed with him is making
you hyperventilate, but just because he's smiling
at you it doesn't mean he wants you, and if he
did, what then? You're not into casual sex, remember.*

*No, but I'd be prepared to make an exception
for this man,* her body sighed as Seth's shirt got
tighter and she felt a warm heat spreading
through her stomach which had nothing to do
with the coffee.

Yeah, right, her brain jeered. *Big talk from a
woman who was a virgin when she got married.
Your life hasn't exactly been a walk on the wild
side, has it, so what could you offer a man like
Seth that he hasn't had probably hundreds of
times before, and considerably better?*

'Something wrong?'

Seth's eyes were on her, puzzled, curious, and
she managed a smile. 'Just thinking.'

'Dangerous occupation, thinking,' Jerry observed. 'A person can get into all sorts of trouble doing that.'

Tell me about it, Olivia thought ruefully. She
uncurled her legs and stood up. 'I have to go.
I've a meeting with Admin in fifteen minutes.'

'Is it about the whiteboard?' Seth said hopefully, and she shook her head.

'I told you before, that it wasn't my deci-sion—or even theirs—to take it down. It's a county-wide ruling.'

'It's still a stupid one,' he muttered, and she nodded.

'I agree, but there's nothing I can do about it.' She carried her coffee-cup across to the sink, then cleared her throat awkwardly. 'I thought I might ask if we could have the waiting room redecorated.'

She waited for the eruption to come, but it didn't. Seth simply shook his head and said, 'If you can screw any money out of Admin, I'd vote for spending it on some new medical equipment.'

'I don't think it's a question of either-or,' she protested, and a wry smile curved his lips.

'Then you don't know Admin. A and E ranks somewhere around the level of Chiropody when it comes to funding.'

Why hadn't he told her that before? She wouldn't have chewed his head off if he'd only told her that before. Slowly she rinsed her cup, then came to a decision. 'Make me a list of ev-erything you think the department needs.'

Seth put down his coffee-cup with a clatter. 'Are you kidding?'

She smiled. 'There's two things I never joke about. Departmental funding and religion.' She checked her watch. 'My meeting's at two o'clock and I need to collect some papers from my office. You've ten minutes to draft a list. If you haven't finished by the time I get back...'

'I'll be finished,' he replied, tearing a sheet of paper from his notebook, and she laughed and shook her head as she went out the door.

Jerry didn't laugh. He sat back in his seat and stared at Seth thoughtfully. 'Told you she was nice, didn't I?'

'Hmm?'

'Olivia. I said she was nice.'

'So you did,' Seth murmured, his pen flashing across the sheet of paper.

'And I think she likes you.'

Seth glanced up. 'Forget it, Jerry.'

The specialist registrar looked innocent. 'Forget what?'

'The matchmaking.'

'I'm not—'

'Yes, you are,' Seth said firmly, 'and there's no way on God's earth that I'm ever going to ask Olivia Mackenzie out. Number one, she's my boss and I've no intention of dating my boss. Number two, she's already in a relationship and I don't poach other men's women.'

'Yes, but— Oh, blast,' Jerry groaned as his pager went off. 'Why do I never get to finish either an argument or a coffee?'

'Think of the good it's doing your heart and your arteries.' Seth grinned, but his smile disappeared when the specialist registrar had gone.

Jerry meant well—he knew he did—but there was a third and even more important reason why he would never ask Olivia out. It was obvious that she was a settling-down sort of a woman, and he didn't want to settle down—not now, not ever.

OK, she was attractive, with the kind of thick curly brown hair that made a man's fingers itch to release it from the confines of the scrunchie she always wore, and she had a pair of soft luminous brown eyes which occasionally made him forget what he'd been about to say, but settling down was for the brain dead. Settling down meant the end of freedom, the end of excitement, the end of everything.

'Have you finished your list?'

He glanced over his shoulder. Olivia was standing in the doorway of the staffroom, her hair gleaming like a halo in the late September sunlight, and for a weird second he felt an inexplicable tightening in his throat.

'Seth, I said, have you—?'

'I...I've come up with eight suggestions,' he interrupted, pulling himself together quickly.

'Only eight?'

Oh, damn, now she was smiling at him. Smiling that smile he hadn't seen since the day he'd first met her, and for a moment he wondered if it would be such a mistake to ask her out. She was single, he was single. OK, she had a George, but...

She's home-made bread, and you're Japanese sushi. She's self-catering holidays with the kids in Cornwall, and you're sky-diving in Brazil. She may have great legs and a sensational smile, but those are lousy reasons for getting involved with a settling-down sort of woman. Especially when that settling-down sort of woman is also your boss.

'I was only joking, Seth.'

Concern had replaced the amusement on her face, and he forced a smile. 'I was just wondering what else I could add,' he lied, and saw her smile return.

'Don't push your luck.' She scanned the sheet of paper and let out a low whistle. 'Seth, these are all very expensive pieces of equipment.'

'I know, but just because the Belfield is old that doesn't mean our patients shouldn't have the best available facilities.'

'Agreed.' She read through the list again. 'I'll do my best, but—'

'Don't hold your breath.'

He wouldn't, he thought as she hurried away, but if anybody could persuade Admin to part with some cash it would be her. She'd just have to look at them with those big brown eyes and smile that particular smile, and they'd be putty in her hands.

He wondered why her husband hadn't been putty in her hands. She didn't strike him as the sort of woman to play around, so it had to be her husband who'd walked, but what kind of lame-brain would walk away from a woman like Olivia? She was attractive, and smart, and her legs…

I thought you weren't going to think about her legs?

He wasn't, he told himself as he drained his coffee and headed for the examination room. In fact, he was going to forget she even had legs, but he was going to keep reminding himself that she had a George.

'Hello, stranger,' Babs said when she saw him. 'I was just about to send out a search party for you.'

'Lunch took longer than usual.' He glanced up to where the whiteboard should have been and scowled at the empty space. 'Right, what exciting, challenging patients can you tempt me with this afternoon?'

'Actually—and I know I'm going to deeply regret saying this—all I can offer you is a swollen finger, two constipation sufferers and a psychiatric patient who says the end of the world is scheduled for three o'clock today and he'd like to build us an ark.'

'Right.' Seth stared at the blank space on the wall again. 'What are Jerry and Tony doing?'

'Jerry has a dog bite in 2, and Tony's examining a Mrs Dickson with stomach pains in 4.'

'I think I'll assist Tony.'

'Thought you might.'

'Hey, I'm supposed to supervise him,' Seth protested, and Babs grinned.

'So how come you only do it on days when you've got somebody who thinks he's Noah as an alternative?'

'Because I'm not as green as I'm cabbage-looking,' he replied, and the sister laughed as he strode across to cubicle 4.

'I think Mrs Dickson has gallstones,' Tony said when Seth joined him. 'There's no sign of any jaundice, but she has all the other classic symptoms. Middle-aged, overweight, high blood pressure and pain in her stomach after she's eaten.'

It was on the tip of Seth's tongue to point out that the last time Tony had commented on somebody's 'classic' symptoms his diagnosis had been completely wrong, but he decided against it.

'Have you had this pain for some time, Mrs Dickson?' he asked gently.

'Three months, Doctor. I thought it was just indigestion, but this morning the pain had moved to my shoulder and I thought...' Mrs Dickson stared up at him with frightened, pain-filled eyes. 'They're always talking in the papers about shoulder pain, how it can mean—'

'Her ECG didn't show any sign of myocardial infarction,' Tony interrupted, 'so I don't think she's had a heart attack.'

Neither did Seth, but as Mrs Dickson whitened still further it occurred to him that Tony's bedside manner could do with a little work.

'I'm sure you haven't had a heart attack, Mrs Dickson,' he said firmly. 'Have you arranged an ultrasound scan to see if she does have gallstones?' he continued, turning to Tony.

The junior doctor nodded. 'The technician's on his way.'

'But I can't have gallstones,' Mrs Dickson protested, wincing as she tried to lever herself upright. 'I never eat any fried food.'

Seth smiled. 'Fried food's not the culprit, Mrs Dickson. It's too much cholesterol. You see, your liver creates something called bile which helps your body to digest fat,' he continued, seeing the woman's puzzled expression. 'If you eat too much cholesterol—fatty things like chocolate, pastries, butter—the excess cholesterol turns the bile into crystals, and it's these crystals that form gallstones.'

'If...if I do have gallstones, will I have to have an operation?' Mrs Dickson asked uncertainly.

Deliberately Seth said nothing, and waited to see what Tony would suggest.

'A course of antibiotics and a low-fat diet is often enough to solve the problem,' the junior doctor said. 'Sometimes we have to remove the gall bladder but it doesn't usually cause any difficulties. Most people can live quite healthily without one.'

Tony was right. He was also a committed, enthusiastic junior doctor, and yet Seth couldn't like him. It had nothing to do with his mistake over the malaria case or even his bedside manner. It was just something about him—something Seth couldn't quite put his finger on—that niggled at him, setting vague alarm bells ringing in his head.

Bells which probably suggested nothing more sinister than envy, Seth thought with a rueful smile as he watched Tony greet the ultrasound technician, then bounce quickly round the trolley to speak to Mrs Dickson. No matter how many hours the junior doctor worked, he always seemed to be full of energy and enthusiasm, whereas he himself...

With a sigh he slipped out of the cubicle. Maybe it was time for him to move on. Time to seriously investigate the possibility of joining a cruise ship or Médicins sans Frontiéres. He'd come straight from med school to the Belfield Infirmary twelve years ago, and twelve years was a long time to work in the same place. Maybe it was too long.

'What's up?' Jerry asked when he saw him, and Seth shook his head.

'I was just thinking about my future.'

'Oh, lord, you're not back to cruise ships and Médicins sans Frontiéres, are you?'

'Something like that,' Seth murmured. 'I just... Jerry, do you sometimes find that young Tony sets your teeth on edge?'

'Of course he does. He's a typical irritating junior doctor.'

'I suppose so,' Seth said, then his forehead cleared as the examination-room door opened and Olivia appeared. 'How did you get on with the big boys upstairs?'

She pulled a face. 'Not very well. I only managed to get them to agree to two of the items you wanted.'

'*Two?*'

'I know it's pathetic—'

'Olivia, I honestly didn't think you'd get them to agree to *anything*.' He beamed. 'What did they OK?'

'The 12-lead ECG machine and the overhead X-ray equipment.'

He stared at her in disbelief. The new 12-lead ECG machines were wonderful. Not only could they diagnose the type of infarct—the blockage in an artery—but they could also detect the severity. And as for the overhead X-ray equipment... For years he'd had to stand by in frustration as their patients were either hauled off to the X-ray department or left waiting until a technician could wheel in the cumbersome bedside equipment. Now their patients could stay right where they were, and because the films were computerised they could be brought up onto a screen in minutes.

'Are you serious?' he said faintly. 'We really can have a 12-lead ECG machine and the overhead X-ray equipment?'

She smiled. 'There are two things I never joke about—'

'Departmental funding, and politics.' He laughed, and without thinking he caught her by the waist and swung her round in his arms. 'Oh, Olivia, I am so pleased I could *kiss* you!'

Now, why the hell had he said that? he wondered as he gazed down into her startled face. He hadn't meant to—hadn't meant it. He'd just been so delighted to hear about the equipment and now he was holding her, and to his surprise she didn't feel skinny at all but warm, and lush, and soft...

'Seth, could you put me down, please?'

A faint tinge of colour was darkening her cheeks, and he watched with fascination as it crept across her face like the blush on the petals of a rose. He couldn't remember the last time he'd seen a woman blush, but Olivia was most definitely blushing. Blushing, and staring up at him, her brown eyes large and dark, her lips slightly parted, and—

'Seth, could you *please* put me down?'

For a second he stared at her blankly, then suddenly realised what she'd said. 'Right. Sorry. I just...I guess I got a bit carried away.'

'We noticed,' Jerry said with a smile that made Seth want to throttle him.

Hell, all he'd done had been to whirl Olivia around in his arms. It wasn't as though he'd done something really dumb, like kissed her. Now, that would have been stupid. Really stupid.

'RTA five minutes,' Babs called from the bottom of the examination room. 'Family of three. A ten-year-old boy with spinal injuries, his mother, who's seven months pregnant, and his father who has severe leg and stomach injuries.'

'Phone Gideon Caldwell in Obs and Gynae, alert Theatre and get me six units of O-negative until we can cross-match,' Seth ordered, thanking his lucky stars for the diversion, only to immediately feel guilty for the thought. 'Jerry, you take the father, I'll take the mother and Tony can take the kid.'

'What about me?' Olivia protested as Seth began walking away. 'I'm not here for decoration.'

She wasn't, but right now all Seth wanted was to get her out of the examination room and back to her office. Holding her had unsettled him, and he didn't like feeling unsettled. He was used to being in control, and this new feeling... He didn't like it one bit.

'Who do you want me to assist?' she continued. 'You or—?'

'I knew I'd regret saying we were quiet,' Babs groaned as she bustled towards them. 'We've also got a twenty-five-year-old male on the way who's managed to amputate his left foot with a garden strimmer.'

'Messy,' Olivia exclaimed.

'Which means you'd better attend to him when he gets here,' Seth declared.

Of course it did, but did he have to look quite so relieved that she wouldn't be assisting him? One moment he'd been whirling her round and laughing, saying he wanted to kiss her, and the next he was Mr Frosty. Good grief, it wasn't as though he'd done anything outrageous like actually kiss her.

More's the pity.

No, it wasn't a pity, she told herself firmly. She didn't want to feel his lips on hers. She didn't want to discover if they were warm and gentle, or hot and demanding.

I bet they're hot. I bet they're so hot that when Seth Hardcastle kisses a girl she needs resuscitation afterwards. I bet—

'Something bothering you, Olivia?' Jerry asked curiously.

Apart from the fact that she was burning? She flashed the specialist registrar a bright smile. 'Not a thing, Jerry.'

He didn't believe her. She could tell from the gleam in his eyes that he didn't believe her, and she groaned inwardly. Why did she have to keep on having these lustful thoughts about Seth? She didn't do lust—never had—and even if she did, he wouldn't be interested. She was too dull, too ordinary, too boring.

'Doc, I need help here!'

A paramedic was pushing open the examination-room door with his trolley, and she hurried towards him. 'Is this the strimmer case?'

The paramedic nodded. 'His name's Paul Logan. Aged twenty-five, extensive blood loss. BP 100 over 60, Glasgow coma scale 3-3-5, class 111 shock.'

Olivia wasn't surprised. If she'd sliced off her own foot she'd be in shock, too.

'Cross-match, BP and heart rate?' Babs asked, carefully sidestepping the puddles of blood the trolley was leaving as the paramedic pushed it into cubicle 2.

'As fast as you can, Babs,' Olivia replied.

'What do you want me to do with this?' the paramedic asked, holding out a plastic bag to her. 'His foot's pretty mangled, but I thought maybe microsurgery…?'

The paramedic was right. Microsurgery could perform miracles nowadays, but the most important thing right now was keeping Paul Logan alive long enough to undergo the surgery.

'Did you wrap the foot in moist saline swabs?' she asked as Babs swiftly began affixing three sticky gel electrodes to the young man's chest before attaching them to the wires of the cardiac monitor. 'Sorry—stupid question,' she added with a grin as the paramedic threw her a look. 'Give it to one of the nurses and ask them to put it in ice water no colder than 4 degrees centigrade.'

'BP 60 over 40,' Babs announced. 'And his skin's getting colder.'

Hypovolaemic shock. Paul Logan's vital organs weren't receiving enough oxygen because of his extensive blood loss, and if they didn't do something quickly he could die.

'OK, start an infusion of Ringer's lactate,' Olivia ordered. 'With luck the lactate should temporarily replace the fluid volume and salts he's losing until we can find out what blood group he is.'

With practised ease Babs set up the IV lines, then swiftly took a blood sample for cross-matching.

'BP unchanged, Olivia, and his heart rate's becoming erratic.'

Olivia glanced across at the cardiac monitor. The sister was right. The trace was jumping all over the place.

'Run the O-negative blood,' she ordered. 'And run it fast.'

'Both IVs wide open and running,' Babs confirmed. 'Heart rate still erratic, BP still falling.'

'Don't you dare die on me,' Olivia muttered under her breath as she applied as much pressure as she dared to the arterial pressure point on Paul Logan's leg. 'I don't allow patients to die on me.'

The IVs were running, they were pumping in O-negative blood like there was no tomorrow, but as the minutes ticked by it became increasingly clear that the young man was losing more fluid than they were replacing.

'Where's that cross-matched blood, Babs?' Olivia demanded. 'We're going to run out of O-neg soon and—'

'Need any help?'

She squinted over her shoulder to see Seth standing behind her, and shook her head. 'What this bloke needs is OR, but I don't know if we're going to be able to keep him alive long enough to get there.'

'How much blood have you given him?'

'Too much,' she replied grimly. 'Babs, what's his BP now?'

'Seventy over 50.'

It was up. Not by much, and not nearly enough, but at least it was up. 'Cardiac reading?'

'The same.'

Live, damn you, Olivia thought savagely as she checked Paul Logan's pulse again. Was it stabilising? It felt as though it was, but it might just be wishful thinking. 'Babs—'

'BP 80 over 60...90 over 60...95 over 70— we've got him!'

They had. It wasn't a great blood pressure, but at least it was high enough to send him to OR.

'That was too damn close for comfort,' Olivia declared, rotating her shoulders to ease the knot she could feel between them after Paul Logan had been rushed to the operating theatre.

'Perhaps, but at least that's one we've won today.'

She looked up at Seth sharply. He sounded tired and defeated, and her heart sank. 'The RTA casualties…?'

'Only the boy made it.'

There was nothing she could say. Nothing that would make it any better. They all had to deal with failure in their own way, but sometimes it was hard. Very hard.

'Seth—'

'Sorry to interrupt,' Fiona exclaimed as she hurried up to them, 'but I'm afraid Mary Miller's back in again, Seth. Cubicle 6.'

'How bad?' Seth asked, looking grimmer than Olivia had ever seen him.

'Pretty bad.'

'Who's Mary Miller?' Olivia asked in confusion as Seth strode away without a word.

'One of our battered wives,' the staff nurse replied. 'It's her third visit this year.'

'Her third visit?' Olivia echoed. 'I hope you've called the police.'

'No, I haven't but— Olivia, wait—you don't understand. If you'd just wait a minute—'

But Olivia didn't wait. She hurried down the examination room and into cubicle 6, only to stop dead in disbelief when she heard Seth declare, 'Mary, if you want to discharge yourself you know I can't stop you, but I think you're being very foolish.'

Foolish? Foolish wasn't the word she would have used to describe a woman with a broken nose and a face that was a mass of livid bruises. The only place Mary Miller ought to be going was upstairs to Women's Medical.

'I didn't want to come here in the first place,' Mary exclaimed before Olivia could say anything. 'My neighbour said she was taking me to the chemist to pick up some paracetamol.'

'I think you need something considerably stronger than paracetamol,' Seth said gently. 'In fact, I'd like to admit you, but if you insist on leaving…'

Wasn't he even going to try to persuade her to stay? Apparently not. Olivia's anger boiled over.

'Mr Hardcastle, I'd like a word with you outside. *Now.*'

He followed her without argument, but as soon as they were safely out of Mary's earshot he put up his hands defensively. 'Look, before you go off half-cocked—'

'Half-cocked—*half-cocked?*' she repeated, incensed. 'What the hell do you think you're doing? I know she's within her legal rights to refuse treatment, but the very least you could do is try to persuade her to press charges against her husband.'

'Olivia, I have been treating her injuries now for three years, and it's always the same. ''He loves me—he didn't mean to hurt me. I must have antagonised him.'''

'But—'

'I can't make her go to the police any more than I can make her accept treatment.'

'So that's it, is it?' she exclaimed. 'Your answer is to wash your hands of the situation?'

'No, of course it isn't,' he retorted. 'Look, perhaps if you'd let me get a word in edgewise instead of behaving like a typical over-emotional woman, we might get somewhere.'

A typical over-emotional woman? Olivia wanted him dead. 'Now, just a cotton-picking minute—'

'Can I remind you that I know Mary Miller considerably better than you do?'

'And can I remind you that if you'd got off your lazy uncaring butt three years ago she might not be in this situation now?' she snapped back.

For a second Seth stared at her, his face a mixture of conflicting emotions, then his jaw clenched. 'Right. Fine. I think you've made your feelings about me crystal clear.' And before she could reply he had spun round on his heel and walked out of the examination room, leaving her gazing furiously after him.

How dared he walk away from her like that in the middle of an argument? How dared he just walk away as though she was some air-headed bimbo who had no right to voice an opinion? For two pins she'd like to go after him and tear his character to shreds. For four pins she'd like to do something really grown-up and mature like kick him in the shins.

'Olivia.'

She glanced round to see Jerry gazing uncomfortably at her, and her eyebrows snapped down. 'You want to add something?'

'Hey, I just work here,' he said quickly, 'but I do think there's something you should know. Seth's been trying his level best to persuade Mary to go to the police for the past three years. He's given her the name of the nearest safe refuge, but—'

'Because she won't listen, he's just given up,' Olivia said scornfully, and Jerry's normally smiling face darkened with anger.

'No, he hasn't. In fact, I'd bet my next pay cheque he's on the phone right now, asking the police to pick up Alec Miller for being drunk and disorderly. They'll do it, too, because they like and respect Seth.'

'But the police will only be able to keep him in custody for a couple of days,' Olivia protested. 'Once he's out he can knock his wife about all over again.'

'Olivia, our hands are tied if she won't press charges, and she won't. Seth's said that she and her kids can stay with him until she gets on her feet. He's even offered her money to help her move away from Glasgow, but she just won't listen.'

'He said she and her children could come and live with him?' Olivia said faintly, and Jerry nodded.

'That's how lazy and uncaring he is, Olivia.'

She stared down at her hands and her voice, when she spoke, was muffled, subdued. 'I owe him an apology, don't I?'

'I think you do.'

'Is he still here, or…?'

'My guess is he probably went home after he made the phone call. He looked pretty angry, and his shift was over so there was nothing to stop him.'

She sighed. 'I'll speak to him tomorrow—apologise then.'

'You're leaving, too?' Jerry said as she slipped off her white coat.

'I should have left an hour ago. Poor George must be bored out of his mind by now. I try to take him out as much as I can, but it isn't always easy.'

'Take him out?' Jerry echoed. 'You mean, he's housebound—disabled?'

She looked confused. 'George is a dog, Jerry. An old English sheepdog, to be exact.'

'He is? Why, that's…that's *great!*'

'It is?' she said, looking even more bemused, and then she bit her lip. 'Thanks for telling me about Seth. He and I…' She shook her head. 'I don't know what it is but we always seem to be rubbing one another up the wrong way.'

'But you like him.'

A faint flush of colour darkened her cheeks. 'Of course I like him. He's an excellent consultant.'

And you're falling for him, Jerry thought with a grin as Olivia hurried away. Now all he had to do was get Seth interested, and then there'd be no more talk of cruise ships, Médicins sans Frontiéres or being too old for the job.

'Has our esteemed boss gone home?'

The sarcasm in Seth's voice was plain, and Jerry turned to him guiltily. 'We thought you'd left.'

'Thought, or hoped?'

'Seth, she's really sorry for what she said,' Jerry protested. 'In fact, she's going to apologise to you tomorrow.'

'She can keep her apology,' Seth snapped back. 'If I never see her again it will still be too soon.'

'But, Seth—'

'I'm going home. Home to where I don't have to listen to, or talk to, or think about Olivia Mackenzie!'

But it proved harder to do than he'd imagined.

'Blasted interfering woman,' he told the television as he shrugged off his jacket and poured himself a drink. 'Blasted overbearing female,' he went on as he carried his drink over to the sofa. 'Always jumping to conclusions, always sticking her nose in where it's not wanted. Everything was fine until she came to the Belfield. I had my work, my home…'

What work, what home? Admin passed you over for the clinical director's job, and this flat isn't a home. A home has decent furniture in it, nice curtains, a wife and kids.

'A wife and kids are for the brain dead,' he exclaimed. 'Once a man settles down it's nothing but DIY and the same woman in his bed until the undertakers carry him away.'

Which doesn't mean that a single man has to live in a flat which looks as though he's just passing through.

He let his head fall back against the sofa and stared at his surroundings. Ten years. He'd lived here for ten years and it was still full of the makeshift stuff he'd bought when he'd first moved in. He could buy some decent furniture. He could hire painters and decorators and get that damp patch fixed on the ceiling.

People were always saying that a change was as good as a rest. Once he'd fixed up the flat he could then investigate the possibility of working on a cruise ship or signing on with Médicins sans Frontiéres. He'd start tomorrow. He'd look through the phone directory tonight, phone the decorators tomorrow and…

He frowned as he stared up at the ceiling. Was it his imagination, or was that damp patch on the ceiling slightly bigger?

He shook his head. It was probably just a trick of the light, an optical illusion, a—

A cry of consternation came from him as he realised that the ceiling above him was beginning to bulge and buckle, and he let out an even bigger yell when a torrent of water suddenly cascaded down on top of him.

CHAPTER FOUR

'MY GOD, you were lucky you weren't killed,' Jerry gasped as Seth put his suitcase down in the corner of the staffroom. 'How on earth did it happen?'

'The police think the couple who own the flat above me left one of their taps running when they went away at the weekend. Once their bathroom was flooded there was nowhere for the water to go but straight through my sitting-room ceiling.'

'Your flat must be in one hell of a mess.'

'It is, which means I need a favour. I wondered if I could stay with you and Carol while the builders replace my ceiling?'

'Of course you can,' Jerry exclaimed. 'We've a spare room that's just gathering dust, and you're more than welcome to use it.'

'I might be with you for as long as a month,' Seth said. 'Once the builders have finished I'll need an electrician, a plasterer, a decorator—'

'Seth, it isn't a problem. We've plenty of room and...' Jerry came to a halt as the sound of Olivia's laughter drifted through to them from the corridor outside, and when he spoke again he sounded pensive, slightly abstracted. 'A month, you said?'

'You won't even know I'm there. I'll go out a lot, see some movies, a few shows—'

'I'm sure you would,' Jerry interrupted, 'but I've just suddenly remembered that Carol's parents could be coming to stay.'

'Could be? Well, in that case—'

'Definitely coming to stay,' Jerry said quickly. 'Most definitely coming to stay.'

Seth sighed as he hung up his jacket on the back of the staffroom door. 'I wonder if there's anybody else who could put me up? I could stay in a hotel, but...'

'We're not exactly awash with hotels in the east end of Glasgow, so you could end up miles from the hospital, which would be useless if we needed you in an emergency.' Jerry nodded. 'Can't you rent a flat?'

'Jerry, I'd have more chance of finding the lost treasure of the Incas than of finding a vacant flat to rent in Glasgow in September. All the students are coming back for the start of the new university term.'

'Hospital accommodation, then? OK, bad idea,' Jerry said as Seth threw him a fulminating look. 'When do you want to move?'

'Like now, you idiot. I've got all my worldly goods in that suitcase.'

Jerry gave the suitcase a hard stare. 'That's all your worldly goods? Seth, you need to get a life.'

'Look, if you're just going to make smart remarks—'

'Sorry.' Jerry glanced down at his watch, and swore. 'We'd better get a move on or we'll be late on duty. Leave your accommodation problem with me. I'll ask around, see if anybody has a spare room.'

'Hasn't Charlie in Dietetics just moved into a two-bedroom flat? I could ask him—'

'I'm sure he's already sharing with somebody,' Jerry interrupted hurriedly. 'Look, leave it with me. I know the blokes at the Belfield far better than you do, and you don't want to end up living with the flatmate from hell.'

'I suppose not,' Seth said dubiously as he led the way out of the staffroom. 'But right now I'd be prepared to share with anyone.'

Which is exactly what I'm counting on, Jerry thought with an inward chuckle as he followed him.

'Heart rate 120, BP 150 over 90, neck veins not distended,' Babs declared. 'Possible fractured left femur according to the paramedic, but he's moving all limbs.'

'I'm amazed he can move anything at all,' Seth murmured as he placed his stethoscope on the forty-two-year-old roofing engineer's chest. 'How high up did you say he was when he fell?'

'Eighty feet. He was examining the roof on St John's in Duke Street, and if he'd landed on the concrete path instead of the grass...' Babs shuddered. 'Breathing 40 to the minute, oxygen saturation 85 per cent.'

'His trachea's central,' Seth observed, 'but I can hear definite decreased air entry on the left.'

'Flail chest maybe—multiple rib fractures, ribs isolating a portion of the chest wall?'

'Looks like it to me.' Seth nodded, wincing slightly as he straightened up, and Babs frowned as she handed him a laryngoscope.

'Are you OK? No offence meant, but you've been looking a bit like Quasimodo all day.'

He shrugged, only to immediately wish he hadn't. 'I didn't get much sleep last night.' Not after being hit on the head by a ton of cold water, followed by an assortment of wood and plaster.

'Never mind,' the sister said bracingly. 'We've only got another two hours to go, and then you can go home and put your feet up.'

Except I don't have a home to go home to, Seth thought ruefully as he inserted the laryngoscope blade into the roofing engineer's mouth and began suctioning away the blood and saliva. Jerry kept telling him he was on the case but he didn't appear to be having much luck in finding anything, which meant he was probably going to be stuck next door to Tony Melville in hospital accommodation for a month.

He glanced thoughtfully at Babs. She wouldn't be the flatmate from hell. She was unfailingly bright and cheerful, and...

'Babs, how many bedrooms do you have?'

The sister looked startled. 'Three. One for Bob and me, one for Katie and one for Allan. Why?'

'It doesn't matter,' he sighed, then frowned. 'There seems to be an awful lot of noise coming from the examination room.'

'Want me to take a look—see what's happening?'

Seth considered the suggestion for a second, then a smile tugged at the corner of his lips. 'If it's a mob of rioting yobs, I think we'll let Jerry deal with it.'

Babs chuckled. 'I don't know about Jerry, but I bet Olivia will have it under control in ten minutes.'

She probably would, Seth thought, his smile fading. She was certainly stroppy enough.

She's cute, too.

No, she wasn't cute. Bosses weren't cute. Bosses could sack you, or ask for your resignation, or give you lousy assignments. Bosses were not cute. *Hold onto that thought. Bosses are not cute.*

'Where's that damned X-ray technician?' he demanded, more irritably than he'd intended, as he gently began easing an endotracheal tube past the roofing engineer's vocal cords and down into his trachea to help his breathing. 'You must have paged him at least ten minutes ago.'

'He's probably taking X-rays in Men's Surgical,' Babs replied, moving the trolley of instruments further to one side to give him more room.

'He's *always* taking X-rays in Men's Surgical,' Seth exclaimed. 'Roll on next month when our new overhead X-ray equipment arrives.'

'Is it still going to be installed in one of our relatives' waiting rooms?' Babs asked. 'BP stable, heart rate a little fast but not worryingly so.'

Seth nodded. 'I know it will mean us losing a waiting room, but the technicians can carry out all the installation work without getting under our feet, and once everything's completed we can still use this old trauma room for minor cases.'

'Sounds perfect.' The sister smiled.

It did to Seth as the door to the trauma room opened, and the X-ray technician appeared, looking decidedly truculent.

'OK, before anybody makes any smart re-marks about me coming via Vancouver, I just want you both to know that I'm not in a good mood,' the technician declared. 'I've already had it in the neck from Men's Surgical this morning, so I'd appreciate a break.'

'Wouldn't we all,' Seth observed dryly. 'I want X-rays of the head, chest, pelvis, cervical spine and legs.'

'Why don't you just ask for a whole body scan, and be done with it?' the technician grum-bled, but he took the X-rays and to Seth's amazement they revealed that, although the roof-ing engineer had sustained multiple rib fractures and a fractured femur, none of his injuries was life-threatening.

'All I can say is his guardian angel must have been working overtime today,' Babs said when the roofing engineer had been transferred to Intensive Care.

Seth decided that his own personal guardian angel must have gone on a permanent sabbatical when he and Babs returned to the examination room to find it full of people with bloody noses, black eyes and split lips.

'What on earth's going on?' he said faintly, and Babs shook her head in disbelief.

'I don't know, but if this is a major incident, what's happened to our triage system? It looks like a complete free-for-all.'

'It's not a major incident,' Olivia said breathlessly as she ushered a middle-aged man with a series of Steri-Strips across his nose out of cubicle 4. 'The police were just worried that if they all stayed together in the waiting room, it might break out again.'

'What might break out?' Seth protested. 'Who *are* all these people?'

'Would you believe the guests at a wedding reception?'

'A wedding reception?' Seth repeated as Babs hurried away to find Fiona. 'But—'

'Apparently the bride's mother took great exception to something the groom's mother said. The groom's father waded in with some choice comments of his own, and the bride's mother hit him, and then the groom's brother hit the bride's brother and… Well, it all got a bit out of hand.'

'So it seems,' Seth murmured with a bemused expression. He scanned the assembled throng. 'Which one's the bride's mother?'

'She isn't here. She's in police custody, charged with assault and battery with a bottle of wine.'

'And the groom's father?'

'That was the man you just saw, with the Steri-Strips on his nose.'

Seth shook his head. 'And people say weddings are romantic.'

'They are,' Olivia declared, then paused and seemed to consider what she'd just said. 'Well, they're supposed to be. Two people, deeply in love, wanting to show their commitment to the world—'

'By signing a contract that most of them will break within five years, and the rest will stick to despite the fact that they're miserable as sin,' Seth said, only to mentally kick himself when Olivia winced. 'Sorry. I forgot for a minute that you were divorced.'

'It doesn't matter,' she murmured, but he knew that it did.

He should have kept his big mouth shut about marriage and divorce, and now she looked lost, and unhappy, and it was all his fault.

'Olivia—'

'If we're talking truth,' she interrupted, 'I've just remembered I still owe you an apology. I jumped to conclusions yesterday about Mary Miller, and it was very wrong of me, and I'm truly sorry.'

Hell, he wished she hadn't said that. He'd felt bad enough at having unconsciously hurt her, but now she was apologising to him, making him feel ten times worse.

'I said way too much yesterday as well,' he replied, desperately trying to shift the blame away from her. 'That crack I made about over-temperamental women—it was below the belt.'

'But understandable,' she said. 'You were angry whereas I should have discovered the facts before shooting my mouth off. Can you forgive me?'

Her eyes were fixed on him, large and dark and uncertain, and suddenly his shirt collar felt too tight.

'Olivia, it's forgiven and forgotten,' he said gruffly.

For a second they stared at one another, then she backed up a step.

'I'd better get back to the wedding party,' she murmured. 'We've treated most of the broken noses and the black eyes, but there's an usher in cubicle 1 with a fractured collarbone and a bridesmaid in 5 who was hit on the head by a piece of wedding cake.'

His lips twitched. 'Dangerous things, wedding cakes—all that heavy fruit and icing.'

A small smile creased one corner of her lips. 'This one was certainly was. Thanks again for being so gracious about Mary. I... Well, I appreciate it.'

He didn't as she walked away. He didn't want her gratitude any more than he'd wanted her apology. It unnerved him, made him feel oddly responsible for her, and he didn't want to feel responsible. He didn't want to feel anything at all except anger because she'd got the clinical director's job and he hadn't, but even that anger was fading, disappearing.

'Seth?'

Fiona was gazing up at him curiously, and he dredged up a smile.

'Something I can do for you?'

'I just asked if you were ready for your next patient, but I don't think you heard me.'

He hadn't. Not a word.

Lord, what was happening to him? he thought as he watched Olivia disappear into cubicle 1. It wasn't as though she was even his type. His type was…

Hell, he was even beginning to forget what his type *was.*

He needed to start dating again. If he started dating again, this constant preoccupation with Olivia Mackenzie would stop—he was sure it would. There was a new nurse in paediatrics—Lucy something-or-other. He would ask her out and—

'Seth—your next patient. The elderly man in the waiting room with acute back pain. Do you want me to bring him through, or…?'

Fiona was looking really worried now, and he couldn't blame her. He wouldn't want to work with a consultant who couldn't keep his mind on the job either.

'Right. Fine. Wheel him through, Fiona.'

The staff nurse did, but by the end of their shift she wasn't the only person in the examination room to have noticed his preoccupation.

'It's just not like him, Jerry,' Olivia declared as they walked together towards the staffroom. 'He's usually so on the ball, but today it's like he's on another planet.'

'You haven't heard, then?' the specialist registrar said innocently.

'Heard what?'

'His ceiling came down last night. The couple who own the flat above his left one of their bathroom taps running when they went away on holiday and their floor crashed into his sitting room.'

'Heavens, he could have been killed,' Olivia gasped, and Jerry nodded.

'It's also left him in a bit of a fix. He desperately needs to find somewhere to live for the next couple of weeks.'

'That explains the suitcase in the staffroom.'

'You noticed?'

'Kind of hard not to when everyone kept tripping over it,' Olivia replied, then frowned. 'He's going to find it really hard to get a temporary rented flat.'

'Impossible, I'd say,' Jerry replied. 'I suppose he could stay in a hotel, but the last thing we want is him living halfway across town if there's a major emergency.'

'One of the hospital flats, then?' she suggested. 'I know they're not fancy—'

'Olivia, I wouldn't put my worst enemy in one of the hospital flats. I would have asked him to stay at my place, but...' The specialist registrar sighed heavily. 'Unfortunately Carol's parents are coming to stay so we've no room.'

'Look's like he'll have to settle for hospital accommodation, then.'

Jerry nodded, then his eyes lit up as though something had just occurred to him. 'Unless...'

'Unless what?' Olivia asked, smiling at Babs as she hurried past on her way out of the A and E department.

'You could put him up for a couple of weeks.'

Olivia's head snapped round. 'Me? But—'

'You bought that big old house in Edmonton Road, didn't you?'

'Yes, but—'

'How many bedrooms does it have—two, three?'

'Four, but, Jerry—'

'He's really stuck, Olivia, and all he needs is accommodation for a couple of weeks.'

Yes, but not with me, Olivia thought, staring at Jerry in dismay. Simply seeing Seth at work was enough to give her hot, lascivious thoughts. What would it be like if they lived in the same house?

'Jerry, much as I'd like to help—'

'He's fully house-trained, doesn't smoke and drinks only the occasional beer and glass of white wine.'

Yes, but he was dangerous. Very dangerous.

'Jerry—'

'He's a colleague, Olivia, and you wouldn't see a colleague stuck, would you?'

Not if it was any other colleague, but if Seth moved in he'd be there every evening, in the mornings, at the weekend.

'Jerry—'

'You do have all those rooms, Olivia, and the poor bloke's effectively homeless.'

He was, which meant she couldn't say no, irrespective of how much she wanted to.

'A couple of weeks, you said?' she murmured, and Jerry smiled.

'A month at the most.'

'*A month?* Jerry—'

'You'd be doing him a huge favour, Olivia, and I know he'd be really grateful.'

And gratitude was the only thing she was likely to get from him, Olivia thought as Seth came through the doors of the examination room and began walking down the corridor towards them. She could probably dance stark naked throughout her house and he wouldn't even notice, so why was she getting in such a stew about him staying with her for a month?

'Does…does he know you were going to ask me?' she said uncertainly, and Jerry shook his head.

'I didn't want to raise his hopes. Look, why don't you make him a happy man—tell him he can stay with you?'

Olivia could think of at least a dozen reasons, but none she was prepared to share with the specialist registrar.

'All right,' she muttered reluctantly, 'but you owe me for this, Jerry, and you owe me big.'

'Goes without saying.' He grinned, and beat a hasty retreat.

Olivia wished she could beat a hasty retreat, too, when Seth drew level with her, but with Jerry hovering outside the staffroom, clearly waiting to ensure she kept her word, there was nothing she could do but make her offer.

'Are you serious?' Seth exclaimed with a look that told her everything.

'Jerry said you were desperate,' she said uncomfortably, 'but if you'd rather not stay with me…'

'No. I mean, yes, of course I'd like to—that is, if you're sure?'

No, of course I'm not sure. In fact, I think I've just lost my mind.

'Of course I'm sure,' she said, determined to radiate certainty and pleasure if it killed her. 'Would you like me to drive you back to your place to collect the rest of your things, or do you want to leave them until tomorrow?'

'I don't have anything else. I've got everything with me.'

'That suitcase in the staffroom contains everything you own?' she exclaimed before she could stop herself.

'I travel light.'

Anorexic would have been her word.

'Right.' She waited, certain that he must want to say something even if it was only, How many bathrooms do you have? But the conversation seemed to be over as far as he was concerned. 'Will I meet you out in the car park, then?'

'Fine,' he replied, and she gave up.

Jerry didn't. Jerry was across the corridor like a shot the second Olivia had gone.

'Everything fixed?' he asked, and Seth nodded slowly.

'I guess so, but... Jerry, are you quite sure you asked everyone? The blokes in Haematology, Charlie in Dietetics?'

'It's a bad time of year,' the specialist regis-trar replied blandly. 'A lot of people are on hol-iday.'

Seth sighed. 'It's not that I'm ungrateful, Jerry, but I can't say that living with my boss and her live-in lover would have been my first choice of accommodation.'

'Her live-in lover?' the specialist registrar re-peated with a slight frown.

'This George she keeps running home to.'

'Oh, right. Seth, about George—'

'I'd better go. She'll be waiting for me in the car park.'

'Yes, but before you go, I think there's maybe something you should know—'

'Tomorrow, Jerry. Tell me tomorrow,' Seth said as he strode into the staffroom and retrieved his suitcase. 'My flatmate's waiting, and I don't want to start off on the wrong foot with her.'

Or with her live-in lover, he thought a few minutes later as Olivia drove him through the busy Glasgow streets.

He groaned inwardly as Olivia negotiated the traffic lights at the top of Duke Street. That was all he needed, to play gooseberry for the next four weeks between Olivia and her partner. But on second thoughts maybe it was *exactly* what he needed. Proof positive that Olivia was out of bounds. Proof definite that she wasn't available. With George in the frame all the weird thoughts he kept having about Olivia would disappear. With George in the picture—

'We're here,' Olivia declared as she drew the car to a halt and switched off the engine.

'Here?' Seth repeated. He gazed out of the car window at the crumbling façade of number 36 Edmonton Road, then back at Olivia. 'This is where you live?'

'I know it doesn't look much now,' she said, 'but as soon as I saw it I knew it had potential.'

'Potential. Right.'

'Admin had already told me how hard it was to get rented accommodation in Glasgow, and...' She flushed slightly. 'The truth is, I didn't know whether I was doing the right thing, taking on the clinical director's job, and I thought if I bought a house I wouldn't have any let-out clause. I'd have to stay, make it work.'

He looked at her and then at the house again. 'I hate to say this, Olivia, but I think the sellers saw you coming.'

'It's a lovely house. Well, it will be,' she conceded when his raised left eyebrow challenged that remark. 'I know it needs work—'

'Like demolition?'

'But the rooms are big and airy—'

'Which means they'll be draughty in the winter.'

'And it has all its original wooden doors—'

'Which I've no doubt greatly delight the woodworm.'

'Look, if you want to go back to the hospital and stay in one of the flats, feel free,' she said as she got out of the car and banged the door shut.

'I was just making an observation,' he said, scrambling out of the car after her.

'Then don't,' she retorted, marching up the steps and putting her key in the lock. 'I love it here.'

He wondered if George loved it as he followed her into the wide, high hallway. Maybe George was a DIY fanatic. Maybe he spent every evening hammering and sawing into the long hours of the night. It wasn't a comforting thought.

'Olivia—'

'Hello, George. Have you missed me, sweetheart?'

Seth gritted his teeth and turned, fully expecting to see a man dressed in a red and green checked shirt carrying a power drill, and his jaw dropped.

'This is George?' he exclaimed as a shaggy old English sheepdog raced up to Olivia, his bottom wagging furiously. 'But... He's a dog.'

'Why does everybody keep saying that?' she said with exasperation. 'Of course George is a dog. What did you think he was—a boa constrictor?'

'No, but—'

'You have a problem with dogs?'

'Of course I don't have a problem with dogs. I had one when I was a kid. I just thought...'

'Thought *what?* Look, George is my best friend, not to mention being an excellent guard dog.' George proceeded to demonstrate just how excellent a guard dog he was by leaning heavily against Seth's leg, then sliding slowly down to the floor and rolling over onto his back, clearly expecting his tummy to be scratched. 'Well, he knows you're not a burglar or a serial rapist,' Olivia continued defensively. 'If you were, he would have leapt straight for your throat.'

Seth stared down at George. 'Do you think he could have found the energy?'

Olivia's lips twitched, then a chuckle broke from her. 'OK, so he's a lousy guard dog, but his heart's in the right place. Look, let me show you around the place so you'll know where everything is.'

The tour took quite a while because the house was so big, but by the time they'd returned to the sitting room Seth was dumbstruck at the enormity of what Olivia had taken on. As she'd said, her house would eventually make a lovely home, but it was going to take an awful lot of time and hard work to transform it.

'It doesn't matter,' she replied when he voiced his misgivings. 'I don't have a husband or children, so I've all the time in the world.'

But you shouldn't be struggling to transform this old barn on your own, he thought as he stared down at her. You should have a man here to help you, somebody to do all the heavy work, somebody to take some of the burden off your shoulders.

'Olivia—'

'Is your room OK?' she continued. 'I know it's a bit basic but I've tended to concentrate on my own bedroom.'

He'd noticed. She'd let him have a brief—all too tantalisingly brief—glimpse of her bedroom, and it had been a lovely room, full of stripped pine furniture and scattered rugs, with a huge patchwork quilt covering an equally large bed.

Actually, a very large bed. A three-person-sized bed. The kind of bed a man and woman could have lots of fun in. The sort of fun that involved taking off your clothes and...

He glanced wildly round the sitting room, desperately trying to think of something—anything—that would take his mind off beds. His eyes fell on the fireplace.

'Good grief, what vandal did that?'

'It's awful, isn't it?' she said ruefully. 'I don't know why anybody would want to paint a fireplace purple. I keep thinking maybe I should just have it taken out—'

'But it's cast iron,' he said, knocking on the fireplace with his knuckles. 'Late Victorian, I'd say. All it needs is a few coats of paint stripper and it will look stunning.'

'I know, but there's so many other things in the house I need to do first, and it's really getting on my nerves.'

'I could do it for you.'

Her mouth fell open. 'Do you know anything about paint stripping?'

'Well, no,' he admitted, 'but don't you just slap on the stuff and the paint falls off?'

Her lips twitched. 'It's usually a bit more complicated than that.'

'I could do it for you this weekend.'

'I couldn't ask you to do that.'

'You didn't ask—I volunteered,' he said, and suddenly she smiled at him, that blinding smile he'd seen all too rarely, and he felt his breath catch and lodge in his throat.

When he'd been six years old he'd discovered that his smile could get him anything, but Olivia's smile was different. It was a smile without guile. A smile that was open, and honest, and completely unnerving.

'Does...does that door always squeak like that?' he said more irritably than he'd intended when George caught the sitting-room door with his shoulder as he passed.

''Fraid so. It's another thing on my ''to do'' list.'

'If you've a screwdriver, I could fix it for you.'

'Do you know anything about—?'

'Olivia, it's a squeaking door. How much of an expert do you need to be to fix a squeaking door?'

She murmured something he didn't quite catch, and retrieved a screwdriver from the window-sill.

'Do you mind if I leave you to it and go and change out of my work clothes?' she said. 'I hate smelling of the hospital.'

'No problem,' he replied, but when she'd gone and he began loosening then tightening the door hinges a chill of dismay ran through him as he suddenly realised what he was doing.

DIY was for the brain dead. DIY was for married men who had nothing better to do with their time.

But fixing a door wasn't DIY. It was self-preservation. That squeak would drive him nuts in two days so it made sense to fix it.

And offering to paint-strip her fireplace?

Dammit, he had to do something to thank her for putting a roof over his head. It would be a small thank-you gift, a way of showing his appreciation. It didn't mean that he—

'How's the door doing?'

He turned to answer her, and the screwdriver slipped from his fingers and went straight into his thumb.

'Oh, my lord, are you all right?' Olivia exclaimed in consternation as he let out a yell. 'How bad is it—will you need stitches?'

'It's a scratch, Olivia,' he protested as she hustled him through to the kitchen and pulled a first-aid kit from one of the drawers. 'All it needs is a plaster.'

'It's all my fault,' she said, totally ignoring him. 'I shouldn't have spoken to you—distracted you.'

And you're still doing it, he thought as she took his hand in hers and gently began cleaning his thumb with an antiseptic wipe. Lord, when she'd said she was going to change out of her work clothes he hadn't expected her to return wearing a pink fluffy sweater and a pair of jeans that looked as though they'd been spray-painted onto her.

How did she manage to breathe in them? How was *he* ever going to breathe again? he wondered as she bent over to throw the used antiseptic wipe into the bin, treating him to a glimpse of a round, perfectly formed bottom.

'Thank goodness you don't need stitches,' she continued with relief. 'I'll just put a sticking plaster on, and... OK, how does that feel?'

She was staring up at him, her cheeks slightly flushed, her eyes bright, and he swallowed—hard.

Maybe he could bribe the builders with the offer of double pay if they fixed his ceiling in a week. Maybe he could bribe them to work twenty-four-hours a day, non-stop, and it would be finished in less. But even if he could, he'd then have to bribe the electrician, and the plasterer, and the decorator, and not even Bill Gates had that much money.

'Seth, I said—'

'What's for dinner?' he asked, desperately trying to change the subject.

'You're in luck,' she replied. 'I did a big shop at the weekend so take a look in the fridge, see if there's anything you like.'

Obediently he opened the fridge, and gazed in horror at the neatly packed rows of chill-cook meals. 'Olivia, this isn't food.'

'Chill-cook foods contain all the necessary minerals and vitamins for a healthy diet,' she said defensively. 'They're quick, nutritious—'

'And they taste like cardboard.'

'Maybe they do—just a little bit,' she conceded, 'but, you see, I can't cook, and—'

'You can't cook? And there was me thinking you were Laura from *Little House on the Prairie*.'

'Laura from…?'

'What else have you got?' he continued, pulling open her cupboard doors. 'Jeez, Olivia, I've seen better stocked mouseholes.'

'*Hey*…'

'Pasta, tinned tomatoes, tinned mushrooms, Parmesan cheese. I can make something from that.'

'You can cook?' she exclaimed, amazement plain on her face.

'I may not know anything about fixing squeaking doors, but my mother had four sons and she was determined that none of us would ever have to get married to enjoy a decent meal. Where do you keep your pans?'

'Bottom cupboard by the sink. Seth...'

He wasn't listening. He was too busy dragging the pans out of her cupboard, and she stared at him in dismay.

He was the flatmate from hell. All the way home in the car she'd been praying that she wouldn't do something crazy like leap on him and demand immediate mind-blowing sex. It had never occurred to her that the only leaping she might want to do would be to pummel him senseless.

'Haven't you got a percolator and some real coffee beans?' he asked, holding up her jar of instant coffee as though it were poison.

'There's a percolator and some beans in the top cupboard, but instant's a lot faster.'

'It also tastes like ditch water so we'll be having real coffee from now on.'

He might be, but she certainly wouldn't, she thought as he retrieved the percolator. A month.

She'd asked him to stay with her for a month. How on earth was she going to stand it?

'I'll go shopping tomorrow—buy some proper food,' he continued, tossing some pasta into a pot. 'Is there anything you don't like?'

Apart from you at the moment? 'Seafood. I like fish, but I can't stand prawns, or shrimps, or anything like that.'

'Really?' He sounded surprised. 'OK, no seafood. What about Indian?'

'Love it,' she murmured, and he smiled. A wide, warm smile that made her heart clutch and her legs feel as though all of the bones had just been surgically removed.

It was going to be a very long month indeed.

CHAPTER FIVE

'So, it's working out all right, then?' Jerry asked as he and Olivia stood at the top of the examination room. 'You and Seth living together?'

'We're hardly living together,' she protested, annoyingly aware that the heat she could feel creeping across her cheeks undoubtedly suggested otherwise. 'Seth's only staying with me because he's got nowhere else to go, and as he only moved in last night it's far too early to tell.'

Except that it wasn't, Olivia thought, cringing inwardly as she saw Seth coming out of cubicle 2. Last night he'd amused her, then he'd irritated her, and then, just when she'd felt like hitting him, he'd smiled. His wonderful toe-curling smile. And she'd gone to bed to dream the kind of dreams that would have been banned by the censors. But this morning...

This morning she'd made a complete and utter fool of herself.

She only had herself to blame. She should have remembered Seth was in the house, but she'd never been a morning person so she'd stumbled out of bed and staggered along the hall, completely forgetting there was a very strong possibility that they would converge on the bathroom at the same time.

'After you,' she'd mumbled, coming to an abrupt halt, all too embarrassingly aware that her hair was unbrushed and she was wearing a pair of ancient pyjamas with little pink elephants on them.

'No, after you,' Seth had muttered back, his eyes flicking to the wall, to the floor, to any-where but her.

'No, really,' she'd insisted, trying desperately hard not to stare, but it was very hard not to stare when you had somebody like Seth Hardcastle standing inches away from you, wearing nothing but a pair of royal blue boxer shorts and a stunned expression.

'I...I'll come back later,' he'd murmured, grabbing the towel off the radiator and holding it against him as he backed up a step.

'No, honestly, it's OK,' she'd protested, backing up, too, and they would probably still have been arguing the point if he hadn't settled the matter by beating a hasty retreat back into his bedroom, leaving her hyperventilating against the wall. Hyperventilating, and cursing herself for being so stupid as to be wearing those pyjamas in the first place.

No wonder he hadn't been able to look her in the face. He'd probably been too busy trying hard not to laugh.

Well, she might not be his type, but she was damned if he was going to think she was some sort of anally retentive little orphan Annie. If she found time today she was going out to buy some new pyjamas. Pretty ones. Adult ones. Pyjamas which made her look like a woman instead of a refugee from a kids' slumber party.

'Possible CVA on the way, Olivia,' Fiona called from the bottom of the examination room. 'Male, aged thirty-five, name of Richard Craig. Collapsed at his home, and the paramedics say his wife's hysterical.'

She was. In fact, it took all of Olivia's powers of persuasion to convince Mrs Craig that she would be better off in one of the relatives' waiting rooms than getting under everyone's feet in the examination room.

'Definite stroke, I'd say,' Seth observed after he and Olivia had finished examining Richard Craig. 'Slurred speech, decreased vision, pronounced muscle weakness with no sensation down his right side.'

'I'll arrange an MRI head scan to define the location and extent of the stroke, and an ECG in case he has any underlying heart disorder,' Olivia replied. 'He's too young to have hardening of the arteries so he could have suffered an embolism—a blood clot which has travelled from his heart to his brain.'

'Yes.'

Something about Seth's tone had her glancing up at him with a slight frown. 'You don't think he's had a cardiac embolism?'

'I think he probably has, but what I'm more interested in is the white powder on the sleeve of his jacket.'

'White powder?' she echoed. 'I didn't notice any white powder.'

'Left sleeve, just above the cuff. It was just a trace, but I'd bet my next pay cheque it was cocaine.'

'You think he's a user?'

'I'd say it was a pretty safe bet, and it's probably what caused his embolism.'

'The idiot!' Olivia exclaimed in exasperation, and Seth nodded grimly.

'I'm afraid there's a lot of them about. Do you want to talk to his wife, or will I?'

'I think this is a two-person job.'

It was.

'How dare you suggest my husband takes drugs?' Mrs Craig exclaimed, her cheeks bright red. 'Richard's a member of the local Rotary Club, he's a stockbroker—'

'Mrs Craig, we're not here to make judgements,' Olivia said gently. 'We're here to help your husband, and if you don't tell us the truth—'

'I *am* telling the truth,' the woman protested, her cheeks darkening still further. 'Richard may have taken the odd amphetamine in the past— just to keep himself going at stressful times— but he doesn't take drugs.'

Olivia glanced across at Seth, and he cleared his throat. 'So, if we send those traces of white powder we found on his jacket to the lab, they're going to turn out to be nothing more sinister than talcum powder?'

For a long moment Mrs Craig said nothing, then she drew a shuddering breath. 'He only takes it because he works such long hours, and it gives him a boost, keeps him alert.'

Olivia sighed inwardly. It was what all cocaine users said, but the trouble was that the effects only lasted for a short time, leaving the user wanting more and more to sustain the high.

'Didn't your husband know that cocaine addicts stand a much higher risk of having a heart attack or a stroke?' Seth asked, and Mrs Craig looked outraged.

'My husband's not an addict. He's not like these down-and-outs you see in the street. He only took it to give himself a bit of a lift, the same way everybody does.'

'Mrs Craig—'

'When will he be able to leave?' Mrs Craig interrupted. 'Go back to work?'

Seth's eyes met Olivia's and she stretched out and took Mrs Craig's hand in hers. 'I don't think you fully understand the seriousness of the situation, Mrs Craig. Your husband's had a massive stroke. He may never work again.'

'But he *has* to go back to work,' Mrs Craig insisted. 'We've just bought a new house, and if Richard can't work we'll never be able to meet the mortgage repayments.'

Olivia stared at the woman in disbelief. If Richard Craig had been her husband, the last thing she'd be worrying about would be a house. Seth clearly thought the same because he got abruptly to his feet.

'We've transferred your husband to Intensive Care, Mrs Craig. I'll ask one of the nurses to show you the way.'

'Not exactly full of the milk of human kindness, is she?' Olivia said after Mrs Craig had gone.

'I predict that Mrs Craig is shortly going to become the *ex*-Mrs Craig,' Seth replied dryly as they walked back into the examination room. 'And the damnable thing is, his stroke's so unnecessary. Why won't people realise that they're dicing with death every time they take drugs?'

'Who's taking drugs?' Tony asked, overhearing them.

'One of our patients,' Seth explained. 'But, of course, according to his wife, he's not an addict. Addicts are the down-and-outs, the unfortunates who live on the streets.'

'They generally are, though, aren't they?' Tony said uncertainly, and Seth sighed.

'Tony, who were these down-and-outs before they hit rock bottom? They were probably people just like you and me. People with good jobs, homes and families. It's a very small step from taking something as a pick-me-up to complete, full-blown addiction.'

The junior doctor said nothing, and Olivia smiled at him encouragingly. 'Don't let the stupidity of the general public get you down, Tony. We can give them the facts, but we can't live their lives for them. All we can do is pick up the pieces for them when their lives go pear-shaped.'

His life had gone pretty pear-shaped recently, Seth thought as the day wore on in a seemingly endless depressing succession of both minor and major injuries. In fact, his life had taken an almighty nose dive ever since last night when he'd moved into number 36 Edmonton Road.

It had been bad enough discovering that Olivia liked to wear the kind of jeans guaranteed to give a man a heart attack, but when he'd met her this morning in the hallway... Lord, didn't she realise how sexy her pyjamas were?

He did. He'd been all too acutely and painfully aware of just how sexy her pyjamas were, and if he hadn't grabbed a towel and beaten a very hasty retreat there would have been two extremely embarrassed people standing outside her bathroom.

He'd have to buy a dressing-gown. If he was going to keep meeting her in the early morning, and she was going to keep wearing those damn pyjamas, he needed a dressing gown. One of those heavy-duty striped efforts that covered everything. In fact, maybe he ought to go for broke and buy some seriously thick pyjamas or a nightshirt. No, not a nightshirt. A nightshirt would leave his legs bare, and he didn't want any part of his anatomy bare. Not if he was going to keep walking into Olivia first thing in the morning.

'Cheer up—it may never happen.'

He glanced over his shoulder to see Jerry smiling at him, and shook his head. 'It already has.'

'Olivia?' the specialist registrar hazarded, and Seth nodded.

'Jerry, she wears pyjamas covered in little pink elephants.'

'And?' the specialist registrar exclaimed, looking distinctly bemused, and Seth groaned inwardly.

Jerry was right. Pyjamas covered with little pink elephants were not sexy. Very tight jeans were sexy, but anybody who thought pyjamas covered with little pink elephants were sexy was in a whole lot of trouble.

'Seth, about these pyjamas—'

'Jerry, do you know anything about squeaking doors?' he said, deliberately changing the subject. 'Olivia's sitting room door squeaks like crazy, and I tried fixing it last night by unscrewing the hinges but it didn't work.'

'You unscrewed a door?'

'Pay attention, Jerry,' Seth said impatiently as the specialist registrar stared at him. 'Yes, I unscrewed a door, and Olivia says I should have used oil.'

'She's right, but… Seth, are you sure you're OK? All this talk about pyjamas and squeaking doors—'

'Oh, damn, and I've just remembered I've got to pick up some food before I go back to Edmonton Road tonight. Salmon would be good, don't you think? And if I cook some courgettes and roasted potatoes—'

'You're cooking?' Jerry interrupted faintly. '*You* are cooking?'

'Jerry, if you saw what this woman keeps in her fridge, you'd be cooking, too,' Seth exclaimed. 'I tell you, she needs a minder. She's bought a house that's falling to bits, she can't cook, and—'

'She wears pyjamas with pink elephants. Seth—'

'Code blue!' Tony suddenly yelled from cubicle 4. 'I've got a code blue!'

For a second nobody moved and then every member of staff who wasn't involved in a critical procedure converged on cubicle 4.

'What happened?' Seth demanded as Fiona swiftly inserted an IV line into the arm of the elderly lady lying motionless on the trolley while Olivia and Babs began performing cardiopulmonary resuscitation.

'I don't know,' Tony exclaimed, his face white with shock. 'Her daughter brought her in because she was experiencing breathing difficulties. I was sounding her chest, and suddenly...' He shook his head. 'She just stopped breathing.'

'Name—age?' Seth demanded, squeezing past Fiona who was attaching cardiac electrodes to the old lady's chest. 'Any history of heart disease?'

'Macmillan... H-her name's Grace Macmillan,' Tony stammered. 'She's eighty-eight, and there was no mention of heart disease in the notes her daughter brought in, but... Seth, she was talking to me, telling me all about her grandchildren—'

'No pulse,' Olivia exclaimed, 'and the cardiac monitor's showing ventricular fibrillation.'

Which meant that blood wasn't flowing from Mrs Macmillan's heart to her brain, and if they didn't get it started soon, the elderly lady would die.

'Give me the paddles,' Seth ordered, and quickly Tony rubbed some conducting gel onto the paddles of the defibrillator and handed them to him. 'Two hundred joules, Babs. Right, everyone stand clear.'

Obediently they all stepped back from the trolley, and when Seth placed the paddles on either side of the elderly lady's chest her body arched and convulsed as the electricity surged through her.

'No change,' Olivia announced. 'Flat tracing, no pulse.'

'OK, Babs, up the voltage to 300 joules.'

The sister turned the dial on the defibrillator higher and Olivia tried not to watch, but her eyes kept being dragged back to the frail figure lying on the trolley.

What kind of life would Mrs Macmillan have if she survived this? She could hear the sound of the old lady's ribs cracking as her body arched upwards yet again, could see the wires in her neck, the tubes in her throat and arms, and she desperately wanted to shout, Just let her go, let her die in peace! But she knew she couldn't. This was what they were trained for, to do everything in their power to keep people alive, so it had to be done, no matter how awful it was to watch.

Still there was no pulse and Seth ordered the voltage to be increased yet again, but when the heart monitor remained resolutely flat at 360 joules he threw down the paddles.

'OK, that's enough. Babs, disconnect all the hardware. Tony, can I see the notes her daughter gave you?'

With an ashen face the junior doctor handed them to him.

'Seth, you did all you could,' Olivia murmured as she saw his jaw clench while he read the notes. 'She was eighty-eight. It was a good age, and her family wouldn't have wanted her to live on in suffering and in pain.'

'They didn't.'

His face was grim, his voice icy, and she blinked. 'Sorry?'

'Read this.'

She took the notes from him, glanced through them quickly and her heart sank. There, tucked in at the back, was a pink form, ticked and signed six weeks ago. Ticked and signed with the words 'Not for resuscitation on grounds of quality of life.' Mrs Macmillan must have discussed what she wanted done with her GP in the event of something like this happening, and her GP must then have discussed it with her family, and Tony hadn't noticed.

'Seth—'

He wasn't listening. He was already waving the pink form under Tony's nose.

'What does it say there in black and white?' he demanded furiously. 'Read it out to me. What does it say?'

'''Not for resuscitation on grounds of quality of life,''' Tony mumbled, his voice small. 'Seth—Mr Hardcastle—I'm sorry…'

'*Sorry?*' Seth repeated. 'Sorry doesn't excuse your sloppy attention to detail. Sorry doesn't undo what we have just done. We have put that woman through hell, and for what? She didn't want us to drag her back to life. She wanted to die.'

'Mr Hardcastle—sir—'

'Get out of my sight,' Seth roared. 'Just…get out of my sight!'

Tony needed no second bidding. Neither did Babs or Fiona or the other nurses. When they'd gone, Olivia cleared her throat awkwardly. 'Seth, he was wrong not to have read the notes, but he's young—'

'He's not going to get much older in A and E if he makes another mistake like this,' Seth said grimly, and Olivia bit her lip.

'I'll speak to Mrs Macmillan's daughter. Explain what happened.'

'Olivia, she could sue the department. We acted totally against her mother's wishes.'

'I know.'

'I don't suppose we could lie—say she simply slipped away? No, I didn't think we could,' Seth sighed, dragging his fingers through his hair. 'Well, all I can say is good luck, and I'm glad I'm not in your shoes.'

Olivia didn't want to be in her shoes either, but to her overwhelming relief Mrs Macmillan's daughter didn't react as badly as she'd feared. She was naturally shocked to learn of her mother's death, but when Olivia told her they'd tried everything to save her mother's life, despite the express instructions on the pink form, the woman seemed strangely relieved.

'Countersigning your mother's non-resuscitation form is a tough thing to do,' Seth said when Olivia told him what had happened. 'You're always going to be left wondering whether you should have signed it, so in a way—though not in a way we intended or want to repeat—I guess we eased her conscience.'

'I guess so.' Olivia nodded. 'How's Tony?'

'I've no idea, and I care less,' Seth said shortly.

She opened her mouth, then closed it again on what she'd been about to say. 'What say we go home? Our shift ended an hour ago, and I don't know about you but I'm bushed.'

'Snap. I just need to stop by the fishmonger's. Salmon with courgettes and roasted potatoes suit you for dinner?'

'Sounds like heaven,' she exclaimed with feeling, and he smiled.

'OK, let's go home.'

'That was wonderful,' Olivia said as she stared at the remnants of the poached salmon on her plate. 'In fact, that was the best meal I've had in years.'

'Considering what you normally eat, I don't take that as much of a compliment.' Seth grinned, and she stuck out her tongue at him as she gathered up their plates and carried them across to the sink.

'OK, fair point, but one thing I do know. If I ever have a son, I'm going to make sure he knows how to cook.'

'You'd like children, then?' Seth said, stretching round her to switch off the percolator.

At the moment, I'm more interested in the sex that comes before the children, Olivia thought, feeling a shiver run down her spine as his arm brushed against her shoulder. *Preferably immediately.*

'I always thought I would have some,' she replied, suddenly realising he was waiting for her to answer. 'When I was a little girl I believed I could have it all—the career, the husband, the family—but life has a sneaky way of overturning your plans.'

'You've still got time. You're only what... thirty-four?'

'After a day like today, I feel a hundred and two,' she said with feeling, and he laughed.

'In that case, what say we leave the washing-up until tomorrow and have a nice cup of coffee instead?'

'Washing up now, then coffee,' she said firmly. 'I hate coming back to a pile of dirty dishes.'

'Is that a not very subtle way of saying I make a bit of a mess when I cook?' he protested, and Olivia's lips twitched as she gazed at the mound of dishes and pans heaped beside the sink.

'Got it in one, but it was worth every dirty pot and plate. Do you want to wash or dry?'

'I'll wash.'

'Would you like to have children?' she asked as he began running some water into the sink and she picked up a dish towel.

'No way,' he exclaimed. 'I mean, can you imagine me ever changing a nappy or sterilising a bottle?'

'Come to think of it, no.' She laughed. 'Now, if you'd said sky-diving in Brazil or white-water rafting in Canada...'

'You see me as Mr Action Man, then?' He grinned.

In every department. 'Well, you're certainly not the stay-at-home, DIY type, are you?' she said quickly, and he threw her a mock scowl.

'You said yourself that what happened with the door was an accident. And if that's the hospital wanting us back,' he called after her as the phone in the hall began to ring and she went to answer it, 'tell them I'm dead.'

Leaving her answering-machine switched on would have been a more sensible alternative, Olivia decided when she lifted the phone and heard her sister's cheerful voice.

'Liv, you're never going to guess what's happened,' Deborah exclaimed without preamble. 'Harry's just been accepted as a member of the Sunningham Golf Club.'

'Is that good?' Olivia asked, curling up on the settle and making herself comfortable.

'*Good…?* Liv, the Sunningham Golf Club is the most prestigious golf club in Edinburgh. It means Harry's finally arrived.'

I didn't even know he was travelling. 'How are the kids?'

'Harry junior's taken up violin lessons, and Joanne's been awarded her grade 3 in ballet lessons, but I didn't phone you up to talk about Harry or the children. I want to know whether you've met any dishy-looking men yet.'

'Deb, I work all day. The only kind of men I meet are patients,' Olivia protested, only to wince when Seth shouted with disastrous clarity from the kitchen, 'Olivia, if you don't come and help me with this washing-up, you're not going to be getting any cocoa and ginger snaps at bedtime.'

There was a momentary silence at the end of the phone, then her sister cleared her throat. 'Liv, that was a man's voice, and he sounds like he's moved in.'

'He has, sort of. But not in the way you think,' Olivia added quickly as her sister tried to interrupt. 'Seth's a colleague—one of the consultants in my A and E department—and he's staying with me because his ceiling fell down.'

'That's a new one.'

'It's true, Deb,' Olivia insisted. 'He can't stay in a hotel—'

'He's not another freeloader like Phil, is he?'

Seth flashed her a grin as he walked past, carrying two cups of coffee and a packet of biscuits, and she leant backwards over the settle to watch him until he disappeared into the sitting room.

'Liv, are you still there? I said—'

'He's nothing like Phil. He's bossy, and funny, and so sexy that all I want to do is jump on him. Not that I ever would, of course,' she added swiftly as a strangled gasp came from the end of the phone. 'Seth and I—'

'Harry was worried this might happen,' her sister declared. 'He said you'd get post-divorce syndrome. It seems it's quite common for apparently sensible women to get involved with totally unsuitable men after a divorce because they're trying to prove to their exes that they're still attractive.'

Totally unsuitable men, huh? Yup, Harry was certainly right about that. Seth Hardcastle was the most unsuitable man she could think of, but she wasn't lusting after him to prove anything to Phil. She was just lusting after him, full stop. 'Deb, I have to go. Seth's made coffee—'

'He cooks?'

'Up a storm.'

'Liv, I think I should come and stay for a few days.'

Over my dead body. 'Deb, I'm not planning on doing anything stupid.' *And even if I was, Seth wouldn't be interested.* 'You've got more than enough on your plate at the moment with Harry being elected to the Sunnyvale Golf Club.'

'The Sunningham Golf Club. Listen, Liv—'

'*Ciao,* Deb, and give my love to Harry and the kids,' she said brightly, and put down the phone before her sister could say anything else.

'Who was that?' Seth asked when she walked into the sitting room to find him stretched out on the sofa with George draped over his knees.

'My sister. She was just phoning to see how I was.'

'That was kind of her.'

Or nosy. No, that wasn't fair. Deborah did worry about her, and in this case maybe she had every right to be worried, Olivia thought as she squeezed onto the sofa next to George and found herself wishing she could trade places with him.

'He'll have you doing that all night,' she declared, seeing George's eyes roll in ecstasy as Seth scratched his tummy.

'I don't mind. As I told you, I like dogs.'

'So do I,' she said, helping herself to a biscuit. 'I always swore I'd never have one—not while I was working—but...'

'But?' he prompted.

'I was driving through Edinburgh to a meeting three years ago, and George was sitting there, tied with an old piece of rope to a lamppost. I tried to ignore him. I even drove on to the meeting, but when I drove back he was still there.'

Seth's face darkened. 'Somebody had dumped him?'

'That's what the police said, so I took him home with me and said I'd look after him until his owners came forward.'

'Which they never did.'

'Why are people so cruel to animals?' she demanded, her eyes a mixture of anger and distress. 'They give you such love and affection, and all they want is love in return.'

George nudged at her elbow with his nose, and gazed soulfully at the biscuit in her hand. Seth laughed. 'Sure about that, are you?'

'Well, most of the time, I am.' She chuckled. 'But I love him to bits, even if he does only feel cupboard love for me. Phil didn't like him but, then, Phil didn't like dogs.'

Seth frowned. 'And Phil was…?'

'My ex. He said he liked dogs, but he didn't, not really, and he always thought George wasn't a proper dog, just a walking hearthrug.'

Seth glanced down at George who was still lying across his knees. 'He is, but he's a very cute hearthrug. How did you and Phil meet?'

'I decided I really ought to take out some life insurance, so I ticked one of those boxes in the newspaper and he came round to my flat in Edinburgh. He stayed for about two hours, explaining how I wasn't maximising the legacy my mother had left me properly, and how I could triple my assets if I followed his advice.'

Seth leant back against the sofa. 'Why do I have a bad feeling about this?'

'We got married three months later,' she continued, ignoring his comment. 'I thought we were happy, but…' She bit her lip. 'I didn't know about his secretary.'

'His secretary?'

'They were an item before we got married and for the two years we were married they were still an item. By the time I found out he'd only married me for my money there was nothing left of my mother's legacy. I wasn't left destitute or anything,' she added quickly as Seth swore under his breath. 'I still had most of my savings, and my salary, but…'

'Why on earth did you marry him?' Seth demanded as George clambered down off his knees and curled up in the centre of the hearthrug. 'I can see why he married you, but why did you marry him?'

'I'd just turned thirty, and some of my friends were getting married for the second time, and having babies, and I…I was lonely. I know that sounds pathetic,' she continued defensively, 'but I liked him and I thought nobody else would ever ask me.'

'Of course somebody else would have asked you,' he protested. 'You're bright, and attractive, and, believe me, liking a person is a lousy reason for agreeing to marry them.'

He thought she was attractive? Her heart did a rapid tango, and she took a deep gulp of her coffee. 'Liking somebody can be just as important as loving them. It *can* be,' she insisted as he rolled his eyes heavenwards. 'If you have the same interests, the same likes and dislikes…'

'Phil obviously liked his secretary a lot more than you did. Sorry,' he added quickly as she winced. 'That was a rotten thing to say.'

'Perhaps, but it's true,' she murmured sadly. 'Maybe it was me—my fault. Maybe I just wasn't interesting enough or...or exciting enough.'

'Olivia, any man who played around while he was married to you is an idiot.'

'I...um... Thank you,' she said faintly.

Their eyes met, then they both stared fixedly at their coffees, and Seth wondered why the hell he'd said what he just had.

OK, so he'd meant it, and he couldn't understand why anyone would ever want to cheat on her, but, dammit, he'd only moved in with her last night and already he was beginning to feel protective towards her, and feeling protective was not a good idea. It was the start of a slippery slope, and he'd spent most of his adult life successfully avoiding slippery slopes.

'Do...? Would you like any more coffee?' he asked in a desperate bid to change the conversation, and she shook her head.

She was remembering the past. He could tell from the sad look in her eyes that she was remembering the past, and he wanted to reach for her, to give her a hug, but she was wearing those damn jeans again. Those jeans which left nothing to his imagination, and he knew if he touched her he'd be lost.

'Biscuit?' he said, his voice uneven, and as she reached to take one his throat closed.

She was so close, so very close. Close enough for him to feel her warmth. Close enough for him to hear her breathing. She smelt of sunshine and flowers, and as she looked up at him, her eyes wide, her lips slightly parted, he just couldn't help himself. He bent his head and kissed her.

He heard her slight gasp, felt her lips move tentatively under his, and then her lips parted, allowing him in, and a wave of dizzying, pulsing heat flooded through him, sending the blood rushing to his head and the packet of biscuits sliding to the floor.

She was warm and soft and he wanted nothing more than to keep on kissing her, but he knew that he mustn't. If he didn't stop kissing her he was going to make love to her, and then he'd leave—because he always left—and she'd be unhappy, and the last thing he wanted was for her to be unhappy. She was born to be a wife and mother. To have kids, and a dog, and a house with a white picket fence. Not that there were any white picket fences in Glasgow, but...

Stop this, his brain insisted as he felt his body stirring and hardening against hers. *Stop this right now, before you get in too deep.* And with an effort he pulled back from her and got to his feet, narrowly avoiding stepping on George.

'I'm sorry. Really sorry. Very sorry.'

'Seth…?'

She looked lost and confused, and he felt like a heel. 'It's late, Olivia, and we have an early start in the morning.'

Her eyes flicked to the clock. 'Half past ten is late?'

'Well, you know what they say. Early to bed, early to rise.'

And with that he bolted. Without even so much as saying goodnight, he bolted, and Olivia stared at George as he clambered back up onto the sofa to take Seth's place.

'What did I do wrong, George?' she murmured. 'One minute he was kissing me like there was no tomorrow, and the next… Surely I can't be that lousy a kisser?'

But, then again, perhaps she was. Phil had said she was boring and dull after she'd thrown him out. He'd also said a lot of other things she preferred to forget.

'I was sure he wanted me, George. Didn't you think—when he was kissing me—that he wanted me?'

George shook his head, and she sighed.

'You're right. I got it wrong. The trouble is, I just so want him to make love to me. Yes, I know that's crazy,' she continued as George shook his head again. 'I know it would end in tears because he wouldn't stay, but... You see, the thing is, I wouldn't care.'

And she wouldn't, she thought as she put her arms round George's neck and hugged him, but it didn't look as though she was ever going to get the chance to prove it.

CHAPTER SIX

TONY sat on the edge of his seat in Olivia's office looking tense and unhappy.

'Mr Hardcastle thinks I'm a complete waste of space,' he muttered, clearly hoping she might contradict him, but she couldn't.

'Tony, you made a mistake yesterday. Yes, it was a big one, but you have to move on from this—try to put it behind you.'

'I should have read through the notes more thoroughly. If I'd only read through the notes more thoroughly...'

'You should have—but you didn't,' Olivia said gently. 'Learn by your mistake, Tony, that's all you can do.'

The junior doctor tried to smile, and failed miserably. 'This will have to go down on my record, won't it?'

'I'm afraid so.' Olivia nodded. 'But I'm not giving you an official reprimand.'

'Mr Hardcastle would.'

He would, too, Olivia thought ruefully, but Tony was shattered enough without her doing that, and what good would it do? He was an enthusiastic and committed doctor, and to have a reprimand on his record so early in his career would kill any hopes he had of future promotion. Yes, he'd made a mistake, but he was young, and she hadn't forgotten was it was like to be a junior doctor, to be always afraid, always stressed and always mind-numbingly exhausted.

'Tony—'

'I always wanted to be a doctor,' he continued, as though she hadn't spoken. 'When I was a little kid I used to watch all the medical programmes and it was always A and E I wanted to work in, but now…'

'Tony, you're still here—I'm not sacking you. Look, we've all made mistakes. Yes, even Seth and me,' she added as the junior doctor shook his head. 'A and E is the toughest department in the hospital. It's stressful, exhausting and you never know what's coming through the door. A lot of people can't cope—'

'I can cope,' Tony interrupted quickly. 'I know what happened yesterday was unforgivable, but I can cope. I want to be an A and E doctor, Dr Mackenzie.'

Olivia smiled. 'I'm sure you will. Now, stop beating yourself over the head with this. You made a mistake, but it's over, done with, so forget it.' He muttered something that sounded suspiciously like 'Seth Hardcastle won't forget it' but she ignored it. They both knew how Seth felt, and discussing his feelings weren't going to get either of them anywhere. She got to her feet. 'We'd better get going. It's half past ten, and you were supposed to be on duty an hour ago.'

Tony nodded but, as she accompanied him down the corridor and into the examination room, her heart went out to him. The reality of A and E was a world away from its portrayal on TV. The programmes could certainly capture the speed and urgency of their day-to-day lives, but nothing could prepare anybody for the mental and physical exhaustion that came from seeing too many people who were either too sick, or too drunk, or just too plain nasty to get medical care anywhere else.

'I suppose he's been crying on your shoulder this morning?'

She turned to see Seth standing behind her, and shook her head at his lack of sympathy. 'Seth, he's shattered.'

'If I'd made a mistake like that—'

'I'd have bounced you straight out the door.' She nodded. 'But you're not Tony. You're twelve years older than him, with twelve years more experience, so cut him some slack, hmm?'

That he didn't agree with her was plain, but something about her expression must have told him it would be unwise to argue with her.

'Maybe what happened yesterday will quieten him down a bit,' he said instead. 'Make him less lively—easier to live with.'

'You find him difficult to live with?' she replied, puzzled. 'I know he's a little bouncy at times, a bit over-enthusiastic—'

'Olivia, he's like Tigger on speed.'

She laughed, and a smile creased the corner of his mouth for a second, then disappeared.

Her smile disappeared, too, as his eyes shifted away from hers and he stared down the examination room at nothing in particular.

He was obviously as embarrassed as hell, and it was all because of that kiss. If he'd only kept on kissing her last night they would have made love, and she would have been happy with that—hell, she would have been ecstatic—but he'd stopped kissing her, and now there was an atmosphere between them. A tense, awkward atmosphere that had been present at breakfast this morning, and wasn't any better now.

Somehow they had to get over this or they'd be tiptoeing round each other for the next month.

'Seth—'

'Olivia—'

They'd spoken in unison, and she didn't know whose cheeks were redder—his or hers.

'You go first,' he said, and she felt a flare of resentment.

Typical man, always leaving the difficult stuff to the woman. Well, OK, all right. She would deal with this if he was too chicken to do it.

She straightened her shoulders and fixed a bright, I'm-as-chirpy-as-hell smile to her lips.

'Seth, if you're embarrassed about last night, there's no need to be. We'd both had a very rough day, and it was a kiss between friends. A sort of comforting kiss, which meant nothing.' Like hell it didn't. If he'd said, Take off all your clothes, she'd have got them off faster than he could have said, Endotracheal intubation. 'So, let's just forget it, shall we? I mean, it's not as though you're my type, or I'm yours, or...or anything.'

'No,' he said hesitantly.

Look, work with me here, you big dummy, she thought, as he lapsed into silence. *I've given us both the perfect let-out here, so the very least you could do is work with me.*

'You're not upset, then?' he murmured, his eyes meeting hers, then skittering away again fast.

Of course I'm upset, you idiot. I'm upset, and frustrated, and mad as hell, but what good will it do if I say so?

'Upset?' she said, upping her smile so many notches it was a wonder her face didn't split. 'What in the world would I be upset about?' Before he could reply, and she gave in to the temptation she felt to hit him, she strode off down the examination room, leaving him gazing after her in confusion.

A kiss between friends? She thought that was a kiss between friends?

That had been a good kiss. On a scale of one to ten, that had been at least a nine, and yet she'd dismissed it as something small, trivial and unimportant. Either he was getting very easy to please in his old age, or he'd completely lost his technique.

Not that he wanted to get his technique back—or at least not with Olivia Mackenzie. He'd come too damned close to losing control with her last night, and it was never going to happen again. Yes, she was attractive, and her lips had been warm and soft and oh, so tempting, but if he'd made love to her last night he'd have felt so guilty afterwards that he'd have felt compelled to stay and then he would have ended up making love to her for the rest of his life.

It was a terrible thought. Terrible because the idea held a certain appeal, and he wasn't a settling-down man. He was never going to be a settling-down man, so he had to keep control of his libido, and his hands off her, and he could do it. All he had to do was work out a schedule that would keep him out of her house every evening for the next four weeks, and it would be a piece of cake.

'My baby, I need help for my baby!' a woman cried as she rushed into the examination room, accompanied by a paramedic. 'Somebody—anybody—please... Please, help me.'

Seth's heart sank as he hurried towards her and took the limp little body from her arms. He didn't need to see the almost imperceptible shake of the paramedic's head to know that it was already too late for him to do anything. One glance at the baby's blue and puffy face had been enough, but he beckoned to Fiona and together they put in an IV line, slid a tiny endotracheal tube down the baby's throat and linked him to a heart monitor.

'I told the day-care nursery,' the child's mother said, clasping and unclasping her hands together frantically. 'I told them Tommy had a dairy allergy, and he mustn't ever have anything with milk or cheese in it.'

Anaphylactic shock. The minute the child had swallowed the food containing dairy products his throat had started to close, and his heart rate had gone into overdrive. The only way he could have been saved would have been if Seth had been there on the spot, able to administer an antihistamine, but even that wouldn't have guaranteed the child's survival if too much of the allergy-inducing food had been ingested.

'Pulse and heart, Fiona?' he murmured, and the staff nurse muttered back, equally low, 'Nothing, I'm afraid.'

'It was written on his chart,' Tommy's mother continued. 'I made sure they wrote it down on his chart. How could they have been so careless?'

How, indeed? Seth thought grimly as he glanced at the heart monitor and saw nothing but a straight flat line. There'd be a court case, and he hated court cases, but most of all he hated the feeling of impotence and helplessness that always came with losing a patient.

His eyes met Fiona's. They'd done everything they could, but even the wonders of modern technology couldn't revive the dead. Now he had to tell Tommy's mother that they'd failed, and it wasn't a prospect he relished.

'I hate it when babies die,' Fiona said when Tommy's mother was led away to one of the relatives' waiting rooms, sobbing uncontrollably. 'How could it have happened, Seth? If it was written on the child's card...'

'People forget. People get careless. Sometimes they get away with it, other times...' He raked his fingers through his hair wearily. 'Life's never fair, Fiona.'

'Are you coming along to the staffroom for a coffee-break?' the staff nurse asked, and he shook his head.

He wanted out of A and E. Just for fifteen minutes he wanted to get as far away from the department as he could. The hospital canteen might serve the worst coffee in the world, but at least he'd be able to drink it in peace, away from the smell of death, with nobody talking about Tommy or reminding him of what had happened.

He got his wish. The canteen was crowded, but something about his face must have suggested he wasn't inviting company so he was left to drink his coffee alone. It was only when he got up to leave that Charlie from Dietetics approached him.

'You're looking a bit frazzled this morning, Seth,' the technician observed.

'Bad day, Charlie,' Seth replied shortly. 'Now, if you'll excuse me—'

'I wondered if you were looking glum because you're stuck with your boss as a flatmate.'

'Certainly not,' Seth replied, making for the door, but the technician came with him. 'Dr Mackenzie is an ideal flatmate.' Or at least she would be if she'd only stop wearing those tight denims and those damn pyjamas with the elephants on them. 'Now, as I said, if you'll excuse me—'

'I wish you'd told me you were looking for accommodation,' Charlie exclaimed. 'I've an empty spare bedroom and, to be honest, I could do with a contribution to the mortgage. I hadn't realised just how expensive it was going to be, owning my own place.'

'You have a spare room?' Seth repeated. 'But I thought... I was told you already had a flatmate.'

Charlie frowned. 'I don't know who told you that. All on my lonesome, that's me, so if sharing with Dr Mackenzie doesn't work out, you know who to call.'

'Charlie—'

The technician was already hurrying to catch up with somebody ahead of them in the corridor.

'Sorry, got to go,' he called over his shoulder, 'but the offer's there if you're interested.'

Oh, he was interested all right, Seth thought grimly as he walked slowly back to A and E.

He'd been set up. Jerry hadn't asked anybody if they had a spare room. He'd been set up, and he didn't like it. He didn't like it one bit. If he hadn't been set up he would never have known that Olivia wore tight jeans and pyjamas with little pink elephants on them, and he would never have kissed her.

Jerry had a lot to answer for, and he had better make it good.

'I must have misheard what Charlie said,' Jerry declared, all wide-eyed innocence and apparent concern. 'I was sure he said his spare room was taken.'

'And pigs might fly, Jerry. You didn't ask anybody if they could put me up, did you?'

The specialist registrar didn't even have the grace to look shamefaced. 'Well, it seemed stupid to ask around when I knew Olivia had that big old empty four-bedroom house—'

'And you thought you'd do a little match-making,' Seth finished for him. 'Well, it's not going to work, Jerry. I'm moving out of Olivia's place tomorrow.'

'Moving out?' Jerry exclaimed, then lowered his voice when one of the junior nurses glanced curiously at them as she crossed the examination room. 'But where will you go? You said yourself that a hotel was useless, and that only a masochist would want to stay in hospital accommodation.'

'Charlie said I can have his spare room.'

'*Charlie?* Seth, you'll never get a wink of sleep. The man changes his girlfriends as quickly as you and I change our socks—'

'Sounds like a perfect way to live to me.'

'But, Seth—'

'I don't like being set up, Jerry. Come tomorrow I'm out of there.'

'But—'

'Oh, and one last thing, Jerry,' Seth continued. 'If you ever—*ever*—pull a stunt like this again, I'll break both your legs.'

A rueful grin spread across Jerry's face. 'OK, I'll back off, but it was worth a try, wasn't it?'

'What was worth a try?' Olivia asked, overhearing him as she passed. Both men looked suddenly uncomfortable, and she came to a halt, her trouble-sensing radar springing to immediate red alert. 'OK, what's going on?'

'Nothing,' Seth replied smoothly. 'We were simply discussing something.'

'I'd figured that much out already,' she said. 'What I want to know is *what* you were discussing. Jerry?'

'I'm sure Seth will explain,' he replied, backing away quickly.

'But, Jerry—'

'Got to go. We've a full waiting room. The usual Friday prelude to the weekend scrum.'

'But...' She was talking to thin air. Jerry was all but running down the examination room, and she narrowed her gaze as she turned to Seth. 'OK, I'm asking again. What's going on?'

'Jerry and I were just saying what a big difference it will make when we have our own X-ray equipment,' he replied, and she shook her head.

'Nice try, but no sale. Seth, you were looming over Jerry like you were the Terminator or something, so if there's a problem I want to know about it.'

Of course there was a problem, but he could hardly tell her that she was it, and as he stared at her he suddenly realised he had an even bigger problem. Telling Jerry he was moving out had been easy. Telling her the same thing was going to be hard unless he could come up with a really convincing excuse.

We're getting on one another's nerves? Not a wise thing to say to somebody who was his boss.

I'm making your home too crowded? Not in a four-bedroom house, he wasn't.

Distance—location? How close was Charlie's flat to the hospital? He racked his brains, desperately trying to remember, and suddenly it came to him. Thornton Avenue. Charlie's flat was in Thornton Avenue, just round the corner from the Belfield. It was perfect. She could hardly get upset if he told her he'd found somewhere nearer the hospital, and he didn't want her upset. It made him feel guilty, and guilt—when it came to women—was an emotion he was unfamiliar with, and didn't want.

'Seth, for the last time, what's the problem? And I want a truthful answer,' she said impatiently. He opened his mouth, fully intending to spin her his tale about finding a place closer to the hospital, but the words died in his throat.

Hell, but she looked so tired today. Tired, and stressed, and the last thing he wanted was to add to that stress. It would be better if he waited until tomorrow. They both had this weekend off, and if he told her tomorrow when they were at her place, with no prying ears, it would be easier, more tactful, more...

Chicken. So, OK, he was chicken, but he'd tell her tomorrow, which meant that he had to come up with something pretty convincing to fob her off with now.

'We were talking about Tony,' he lied, and saw her bristle, which was better than seeing her looking hurt. 'We were wondering if he had it in him to make a good A and E doctor.'

'I don't think that's for you to decide,' she said tightly. 'You and Jerry are certainly entitled to your opinions, but the final decision is mine.'

'Of course.'

She was staring at him suspiciously. He'd given in too easily—way too easily—and she was no fool. She was going to gnaw and gnaw at this if he didn't find a way of heading her off. To his relief rescue suddenly began walking towards him in a most unlikely guise.

'Whoa, but this looks like a ripe one,' he exclaimed. 'Want to toss for him?'

Olivia wanted to retreat to the fresh air of her office when she turned to see Babs leading a man dressed in the filthiest rags she'd ever seen towards one of the cubicles, but not for one minute would she ever have admitted it.

'I'll take him,' she said, and Seth grinned.

'Why don't we both take him? If the two of us work on him together we'll be able to get him and his interesting aroma out of the department faster.'

A truly independent woman would have said, I don't need help, but Olivia wasn't that independent, or that stupid.

'Sounds good to me,' she said.

It sounded even better when they joined Babs in cubicle 3, and the smell emanating from the man could be enjoyed at close quarters.

'His name's Ronnie,' the sister said, choking slightly as she cut off the man's trousers and dropped them to the cubicle floor. 'Apparently he tripped on the kerb in Duke Street and fell over.'

'Cut me leg a bit, Doc,' Ronnie wheezed. 'So if you could just stick a bit of plaster on it, I'll be out of here in no time.'

Ronnie's leg needed a lot more than a piece of plaster, Olivia thought as she stared down at it. The cut he'd sustained was jagged, inflamed and very angry-looking.

'How long ago did you fall?' she asked.

'A week—maybe ten days ago. Look, Doc, can't you just get on with it? I've friends to meet, places to go.'

Probably the nearest park to drink some methylated spirits, Olivia thought ruefully as she snapped on a pair of examination gloves, then reached for a face mask. She didn't like wearing one, but TB was rife amongst the homeless and Ronnie looked as though he'd been on the streets for years.

'I'll suture his leg, if you want to do a quick physical,' Seth said, and she nodded.

Ronnie might smell to high heaven, and he undoubtedly wouldn't thank her for an examination, but he'd once been somebody's son—perhaps even somebody's husband and father—and if he had any underlying medical condition it was their job to find it and treat it.

'Anything we should worry about?' Seth asked, when she'd finished her examination and he'd finished suturing Ronnie's leg.

'Some crackles in his chest, and his BP's pretty high.'

'You just leave me chest alone,' Ronnie exclaimed belligerently. 'If you're finished with me leg I'll be off.'

Olivia glanced across at Seth, and he shrugged. They couldn't make the man stay or force him to have a chest X-ray.

'I want to give you a tetanus injection, Ronnie. I really do think it would be wise, don't you?' she said as he began to complain. 'The streets are filthy, and you don't want to lose that leg, do you?'

'I don't like needles.'

'I don't think anybody does.' She smiled, taking the syringe Babs was holding out to her. 'All you have to do is relax and—' She let out a small exclamation as Ronnie jerked his leg slightly, knocking her elbow against the side of the trolley. 'Just keep still...keep still... There, it's all done.'

'Dr Mackenzie, could I have a word?'

She glanced up to see Seth staring at her, his face oddly tense. 'I won't be a minute. Babs, could you see if we can rustle him up a pair of trousers?' The sister nodded, and Olivia turned back to Ronnie. 'You'll need to come back in a week's time so we can take out the stitches, but in the meantime—'

'Dr Mackenzie, I want a word with you. *Now.*'

Seth's voice was harsh, insistent, and she followed him out of the cubicle in confusion, but the minute they were standing in the examination room he caught hold of her hand, pulled off her examination glove and stared down at her fingers.

'What are you doing?' she protested. 'Seth—'

'I thought so. You've got a needlestick injury.'

She stared down at her hand. She'd felt the syringe catching her hand when Ronnie had jerked his leg and, sure enough, there on her thumb was the tiniest pinprick, and a small blob of blood.

'Seth, that has to be the crappiest needlestick injury I've ever seen. In fact, I wouldn't even call it a needlestick injury.'

'I would, and that man could have hepatitis C or be HIV positive.'

A chill of fear ran down her back, and she stamped on it quickly.

'Seth, the pinprick is tiny, and even if it was bigger there's only a 0.2 to 0.5 per cent chance that I could become infected with HIV.'

'And a 10 per cent chance that you could catch hepatitis C,' he retorted, and before she could argue he'd marched her across to the sink and began scrubbing her hand with soap and water until she thought he'd take the skin off.

'Seth, you're overreacting,' she protested as he led her inexorably towards her office, then made her roll up her sleeve so he could take a blood sample. 'Look, you can't even see where the needle went in now.'

'Where do you keep the forms we have to sign to get the anti-retroviral drugs for HIV?' he demanded, completely ignoring her.

'In the bottom drawer of the filing cabinet, but—'

'Olivia, you are going to sign those forms if I have to break all your fingers to do it.'

'Big talk,' she huffed. 'I'd like to remind you that I'm in charge of this department.'

'You can remind me all you like, but I'm not the one with the needlestick injury.'

There was no answer to that, and she signed the forms with singularly bad grace, but as he shot out of her office, telling her to stay put, she wished there was an answer. She wished even more that he'd hurry back. It wasn't that she was worried, but...

She stared down at her thumb. She'd been lying. She could still see the pinprick, but she couldn't catch hepatitis C or become HIV positive. People like her didn't. *Yes, they did. All the time*.

'OK, I've got the pills,' Seth declared when he reappeared. 'You're to take the whole course and—'

'Seth, those aren't pills,' Olivia gasped as she stared at the three tubs full of huge yellow pills he was carrying. 'That's horse medicine, and I'll never get them down my throat.'

'I wouldn't worry too much about your throat,' he replied, his blue eyes gleaming as he poured some water into a tumbler. 'It's your other end that's really going to feel it.'

'In what way?' she said uncertainly, and the gleam in his eyes deepened.

'Well, let's just say that not only are you lucky to have tomorrow and Sunday off, but the blokes in pharmacy strongly recommend you take the rest of today off as well, and stay close to a loo for the next thirty-six hours.'

She straightened up in her seat. 'Couldn't we just wait until we find out whether Ronnie has hepatitis C or is HIV positive? I mean, it seems stupid to take something only to find out later that I didn't need to.'

'Olivia, will you stop being such a baby?' Seth protested. 'You know perfectly well that the anti-retroviral drugs for HIV only work if you take them within an hour, and we won't know the hepatitis C results until tomorrow and the HIV results until Sunday afternoon.'

'Yes, but—'

'Olivia, if you don't swallow these damn pills I'm going to force them down your throat.'

She gave him a very hard stare, then took the pills, gagging on the last one as it stuck in her throat. 'Happy now?' she demanded, her eyes watering as she handed him back the tumbler.

'I'll get Ronnie's confidential HIV test organised, and then I'll drive you home.'

'You don't need to drive me home,' she protested. 'I'm not an invalid.'

He grinned at her as he strode to the door. 'No, but if those pills work as fast as the blokes in pharmacy said, I think you might find it difficult to drive cross-legged.'

'You're enjoying this, aren't you?' she said weakly when she staggered out of her bathroom, feeling distinctly nauseous. 'This is payback time for everything I've ever said to you.'

'Would I be that rotten?' Seth demanded, then laughed when she nodded. 'Look, go and put your feet up in the sitting room and I'll make you some soup.'

'I couldn't eat a thing.'

'You may not want to, but it will be better for your stomach if you try. It won't take me a minute, then I'll take George out for a walk.'

She nodded, only to realise suddenly what he'd said. 'You don't have time to take George for a walk. You need to get back to work.'

'Tony and Jerry can manage perfectly well on their own for the rest of today without me.'

'But—'

'Olivia, if there's some mega-emergency, they'll page me, but right now I'm staying here.'

'But—'

'Your phone's ringing.'

She scowled at him, and went to answer it.

'You're there,' her sister exclaimed.

'Of course I'm here,' Olivia replied. 'I wouldn't be talking to you otherwise.'

'No, I meant I expected to get your answering-machine. Shouldn't you be at work?'

'I...I've got a stomach bug,' Olivia lied. 'A bit of diarrhoea. It's nothing to worry about but I thought I might be better at home.'

'Don't stay on the phone too long,' Seth called from the kitchen. 'Your soup's almost ready.'

'Why is Seth there?' her sister asked. 'Does he have the same stomach bug as you?'

'He drove me home because he said I couldn't possibly drive myself. Actually, he was right,' Olivia added ruefully. 'We had to stop twice so I could dash into the nearest loo.'

'Yes, but why is he still there—why hasn't he gone back to work?'

'I think he just wants to see me suffer.'

'I don't. I've changed my mind about him. If you really like him, I think you should go for it.'

Olivia pushed back her hair from her fore-head. Lord, now she was sweating. Sweating, and her stomach had begun to cramp again which meant this was going to be a very short phone call. 'Deb, I have diarrhoea. I do not think that's a big turn-on for a man.'

'So how long do you think the diarrhoea will last?'

Until I die? No, there was no point in telling her sister she might have hepatitis C or be HIV positive. Deborah freaked out if she got so much as a splinter in her finger. 'About thirty-six hours.'

'Then you can hit on him in thirty-six hours.'

She had to be joking. 'Deb, trust me. Even if I took off all my clothes in front of this man, he would not be interested.'

'Liv, he drove you home, and he's staying with you. He's interested. All you have to do is look sexy and jump on him.'

Look sexy. Right. Olivia stared at the wan face that was gazing back at her from the hall mirror, and sighed. Even if she was fit enough to jump on him he wouldn't be interested. Look at what had happened when they'd kissed. She hadn't been the one who'd stopped—he had. She just wasn't exciting. She just wasn't sexy.

And she had diarrhoea, she thought as she bade a hasty farewell to her sister and rushed to the toilet again. Why couldn't she have been sick? OK, so being sick was hardly romantic, but he could have mopped her forehead, maybe held her hand. But diarrhoea... There was nothing even remotely romantic about having diarrhoea.

'Why don't you go to bed?' Seth said when she made a valiant but unenthusiastic attempt at the soup he'd made. 'Maybe if you lie down for a while you might feel better.'

'What's the point?' she moaned. 'I'm only going to have to get up again.'

He gathered up their soup bowls. 'If it's any consolation, the lab said the worst of the diarrhoea should be over in twenty-four hours.'

'I'll be dead in twenty-four hours,' she said bitterly, and he laughed.

'No, you won't. Get yourself off to bed, and I'll take George out for a walk.' She got gingerly to her feet, and his smile disappeared. 'Are you going to be OK on your own—getting your clothes off, and so on?'

A sexy woman would have said no. A sexy woman would have batted her eyelashes and looked pathetic, and then Seth would have helped her out of her clothes, and she could have ended up naked, and…

Felt like a total idiot when he did nothing but help her into her godawful pyjamas. Not that he was likely to make a move on her even if she'd been dressed in red lace. No man in his right mind would want to make love to a woman who kept running to the bathroom. A woman who might have hepatitis C or be HIV positive.

She sniffed, and muttered, 'I can manage, thank you.'

To her surprise he reached out, cupped her chin in his hand and tilted her face up to his.

'Hey, come on, Liv,' he said gently. 'I know you're feeling lousy, but we'd much rather you felt lousy than run the risk of losing you.'

He'd called her Liv, and only her parents and her sister ever called her that, and it was his use of her old childhood nickname rather than what he'd said that brought tears welling into her eyes.

'Oh, Liv, don't cry,' he exclaimed in horror. 'Please—please, don't cry.'

'I'm not crying—honestly I'm not,' she hiccuped. 'I'm just… I'm… Oh, damn, I'm sorry, but I need to go to the loo again.'

Which just about summed up her life, she thought when she eventually crawled into bed and heard the sound of her front door closing, which meant Seth was taking George out for a walk as he'd promised. Everything she touched seemed to go straight down the toilet. The sexiest man she'd ever met was living with her, and where was she?

Alone in bed with diarrhoea, wearing a pair of pyjamas with little pink elephants on them, waiting for the results of a blood test.

CHAPTER SEVEN

SHE slept until eleven o'clock on Saturday morning. OK, so she'd needed to get up twice during the night, and each time George had shot her an irritated look from his position at the bottom of her bed, but she couldn't believe it when she stared at her bedside clock and found that half the morning was gone.

'How are you feeling?' Seth asked when Olivia teetered unsteadily into the kitchen.

'Better,' she said cautiously, not wanting to tempt the gods. 'A bit better. Is there any coffee in the percolator?'

'I switched it on when I heard you coming downstairs. What would you like for breakfast? I could scramble some eggs—'

'Toast, please—just toast.'

And a new face, and a new body, she added mentally as he slipped two slices of bread into the toaster, and she saw he was wearing jeans. Jeans and a matching denim shirt. She'd never seen him wearing anything but a white shirt and dark trousers before and, of course, he looked gorgeous while she looked half-dead. Life was so unfair.

'What's that odd smell?' she asked as the toaster popped and the percolator began to bubble.

'The coffee?' he suggested, stepping over George to hand her the butter and marmalade. 'Those anti-retroviral drugs can play havoc with your sense of smell.'

'Not in here. Out in the hall. I smelt it when I passed the sitting room. A sharp, catch-you-at-the-back-of-your-throat sort of smell.'

'That'll be the paint stripper.'

She put down the marmalade. 'The paint stripper?' she repeated uncertainly, and he beamed, looking for all the world like a small boy who'd just been given a new toy.

'George and I took a walk after breakfast, and we found this paint shop. The owner was really helpful—'

'Morrison's Paint and DIY in Duke Street?'

'That's the one. You wouldn't believe how much stuff you need to take paint off a fireplace.'

She would if it was Ian Morrison doing the selling. Ian Morrison would sell you half his shop if he thought you were mug enough to buy it.

'Seth, are you quite sure about this paint stripping?' she said. 'It's not that I don't appreciate your offer, but—'

'Of course I'm sure. No,' he said firmly to George who had got up on his hind legs to investigate the biscuit jar on top of the worktop. 'You've had two biscuits this morning, so no more. Oh, all right. *One.* You can have one more biscuit, and that's it.'

'You're spoiling him rotten.' Olivia chuckled. 'All these long walks and biscuits. If you keep this up he'll be moving out with you when you leave in a month.'

'It's just cupboard love,' Seth muttered, but to her surprise he looked suddenly uncomfortable, almost guilty.

What had she said wrong? She'd only said the truth, but maybe he didn't like the idea of George getting attached to him. She could understand that. She was a sucker for a pair of soulful doggy eyes, and George possessed a pair of the best.

'Seth—'

'Why in the world did you ever buy this house?' he demanded with more irritation than his question warranted. 'You're going to be working on it for years. Four bedrooms. What on earth does a single woman want with four bedrooms?'

'It wasn't the number of bedrooms that attracted me,' she said, taking a bite from her toast. 'It was the whole house. I'd told the estate agent how much I was prepared to pay, and he gave me a list of possible properties, and the minute I opened the front door I knew I'd fallen in love.'

'Fallen in love?'

'OK, so maybe that sounds a little weird,' she said defensively, 'but, you see, I knew the house needed me as much as I needed it, and that I could make it beautiful again.'

'And do you often fall in love with houses?' Seth asked as he poured her out some coffee and George padded round the table to sit down beside her and stare at her toast.

'Of course I don't,' she said, knowing he was laughing at her but willing him to understand. 'I just... All I initially wanted was a place of my own. I lived with my parents when I was growing up, then I rented a bedsit when I was at med school, and then I rented a flat when I worked at the Edinburgh General. I wanted something that was mine. A place that nobody could ever take away from me.'

'Didn't you and Phil buy a house when you got married?'

'He said the house market was too volatile to make such a big investment. What he really meant was that he'd far rather use the money to entertain his secretary.' Seth's jaw clenched, and she shook her head. 'Sorry, that sounded bitter and self-pitying, and I don't feel sorry for myself, honestly I don't.'

'Why didn't your sister or your parents say something when you got involved with this jerk?' he demanded harshly.

'My dad died when I was in med school—he had a massive heart attack just before my final exams—and my mother died three years ago of breast cancer, so they weren't around to say anything.'

'I'm sorry.'

'It's OK,' she said with an uneven smile. 'I'm not the only woman in the world to have lost both her parents. And as for my sister... Are your brothers older or younger than you?'

'They're all older.'

'And do you take any notice of what they say?'

He grinned a little ruefully. 'No, never.'

'Well, there you are.' She fed George the rest of her toast, then took a sip of the coffee Seth had poured for her. 'It's ironic, really. When Deb and I were small our mother always said that Deb got the looks and I got the brains, but when it came to holding onto her half of our mother's legacy Deb definitely had the brains.'

'She must be some looker. Your sister, I mean,' he continued as she stared at him, puzzled. 'Because you're no cold potato yourself.'

'I... Why...thank you.'

'Don't mention it.'

Their eyes met, and it was he who looked away first.

'I'd better see how the paint stripper's doing,' he muttered. 'Mr Morrison said to leave it on the fireplace for twenty minutes, and I've been doing that but it doesn't seem to be having much effect.'

'In what way doesn't it seem to be having much effect?' she asked, following him out of the kitchen, clutching her coffee, with George padding along behind.

'Well, the paint's certainly coming off, but—'

'Coming *off?*' she gasped as she stopped dead in the doorway of the sitting room and stared in horror at her fireplace. George sneezed and sneezed, then bolted back into the kitchen. 'Seth, it's green now, and orange, and brown, and pink, and—'

'That's only because other vandals have painted it over the years,' Seth replied, his voice a mixture of confidence and uncertainty. 'If it had only been painted purple, it would be finished by now, but...' He stared at the fireplace and frowned. 'I might have to nip down to Morrison's for some more paint stripper.'

Olivia stared at the four empty cans which were already lying on top of a black plastic bin liner, and the heap of paint-daubed newspapers and discarded rags. 'More paint stripper...' And suddenly she couldn't help herself. A bubble of laughter broke from her. 'Seth, I think maybe you should just stick to the cooking from now on, and leave the DIY to me.'

'You reckon?'

'I reckon.' She nodded.

'I suppose you're right,' he said, then his eyes shifted longingly back to the fireplace. 'It's just that I did promise to do it for you, and I've got this far...'

He wanted to finish it. It was as plain as the paint scraper in his hand that he wanted to finish it, and if she agreed he'd probably still be working on the damned fireplace next Saturday, but...

'Of course, when I said you should stick with the cooking I didn't mean you were off the hook with the fireplace,' she said. 'I'm expecting you to finish that.'

'Really?' he exclaimed, and when she nodded he smiled. A wide wonderful smile that had her breath catching in her throat and her heart doing a double somersault.

Lord, but she wanted this man. Wanted him with a passion she had never felt for Phil. He'd made one unholy mess of her fireplace, the house would probably stink for weeks of paint stripper, but all she could think as she watched him get down on his hands and knees beside the fireplace was how hot and sexy he looked, and how much she ached to touch him, to have him hard against her, and deep inside her.

'What?' he asked, looking up and finding her gaze on him.

I want you. 'I was just wondering if there was anything I could do to help,' she lied, and he shook his head.

'All I want you to do is to sit on the sofa and relax,' he insisted, and she did.

They talked about anything and everything throughout the rest of the day as he scraped away at the fireplace, and she ferried him cups of coffee and occasionally—thankfully increasingly only occasionally—made hurried trips to the bathroom. They celebrated with some of his home-made soup and rolls for lunch when the hospital phoned to say there was no sign of hepatitis C in her blood, and he showed her how to make *caffe latte* with a percolator, and neither of them mentioned the HIV result that they wouldn't get until tomorrow.

'Of course, all my brothers are married now, with families,' he said, when the light became too poor for him to continue working on the fireplace. 'I'm the only one who's single, and the only one who was daft enough to choose a medical career.'

'You think choosing a medical career was a mistake?' she said curiously, and he sighed as he slipped a chicken casserole into the oven for their dinner.

'Not a mistake, no, but just lately…I've been wondering about whether I should make a change, perhaps leave A and E and sign on as a doctor on one of those cruise ships.' He frowned as her lips twitched. 'Why does everyone laugh when I say that?'

'Probably because none of us can picture you sailing the seven seas, dispensing seasickness pills and being pursued by the blue-rinse brigade.' She stopped. 'Actually, I take that back. I *can* picture you being pursued by the blue-rinse brigade.'

'You think I might appeal to the over-sixties, then?'

Seth, you'd appeal to anyone. 'If you're angling for a compliment, you've come to the wrong woman,' she said, and he stuck out his tongue at her as he began setting the table. 'But I can understand you wanting a change. I threw up a perfectly good job in Edinburgh to move to Glasgow.'

He paused as he took two glasses out of the cupboard. 'It wasn't just the promotion that attracted you, then?'

'It was partly that, but mainly I just wanted to get away. Away from all my well-meaning friends who kept saying how sorry they were about Phil.'

'And have you had any regrets about moving to the Belfield?'

She shook her head. 'I like fixing things. Taking things—situations, places—that aren't working properly and making them work.'

'And does this interest in fixing things extend to people?'

Only once, she thought, and that had been with Phil, but not even she had been able to fix that.

'No, it doesn't,' she said abruptly.

'I'm sorry.'

She glanced up at him quickly. How did he know? How could he possibly know what she'd been thinking? But she could tell from the understanding and sympathy in his deep blue eyes that he did.

'It's all water under the bridge now,' she said.

'But it still hurts.'

Did it? It had hurt like hell when she'd first found out about Phil's secretary. She'd felt so betrayed, and deceived, and stupid, but now… She forced herself to think about Phil, to remember the things he'd said when she'd thrown him out, and, no, it didn't hurt any more. She'd finally let go of the past and, though he would never know it she had Seth to thank for that.

'I just hope he turns up in our department one day,' Seth said grimly.

'Revenge of the enema?' she suggested with an uneven smile, and he nodded.

'With a fibre-optic endoscopy for good measure.' She laughed, and as the phone in the hall began to ring, and she went to answer it, he called after her, 'If that's the hospital, tell them I'm only coming if World War Three has broken out, and if it's your sister, say hi to her from me.'

It was her sister, full of kindness and solicitude, and completely eaten up with curiosity.

'Forget the children and Harry, Liv,' she said, cutting into Olivia's enquiries without a qualm. 'I want to know what's happening between you and Seth.'

'Nothing's happening, Deb,' Olivia replied.

'Don't be long on the phone, Liv,' Seth shouted from the kitchen. 'Dinner will be ready in about fifteen minutes.'

'Liv—he's calling you Liv now?' her sister exclaimed.

'He only just started, and it doesn't mean anything—'

'You never let Phil call you Liv in the two years you were married so it does mean something. It means you're really serious about this guy.'

Oh, I'm serious all right, Olivia thought as Seth wandered past her, collected George from the sitting room and then wandered back, oozing testosterone and sex appeal, and everything she'd always wanted and had never had.

'Deb, I've had more hot thoughts about this man in the last three and a half days than I had in the two years I was with Phil,' she whispered down the phone, 'but it's no use. He hasn't once made a move on me.' Which wasn't strictly true, but there was no way she was going to tell her sister about the aborted kiss. A woman had her pride. 'Deb—'

'Maybe you're not sending out the right signals.'

'I don't think it would help if I bought a set of flags and spelt it out in semaphore.'

'Maybe it's because you're his boss. A lot of men have a problem with the thought of a woman on top.' A male voice said something in the background, and she heard her sister say, 'Yes, they do, Harry, and this is my sister, so butt out. Liv…Liv, are you still there?'

She was, but she was having trouble concentrating now that Deborah had conjured up an image in her mind of her lying on top of Seth. Of her sliding down over his muscular chest, easing herself onto him.

'Deb, I don't think it has anything to do with me being his boss,' she said quickly. 'Seth Hardcastle is the least insecure man I know. It's me. He's just not attracted to me.'

'Perhaps he thinks it would be wrong to make a move on you when you've been kind enough to give him accommodation,' Deborah said without much conviction. 'Or perhaps he's too much of a gentleman.'

'Not according to his reputation he's not. According to his reputation he's sex on legs.'

'Then there's only one thing you can do. You'll have to make a move on him.'

Olivia choked over the phone. 'Are you out of your mind?'

'Liv, join the rest of us in the twenty-first century. If a woman is interested in a man she tells him so.'

Olivia thought about telling Seth she wanted to make love to him and shrivelled inside. 'Deb, I can't.'

'OK, if that's how you feel, but if I were you I'd just grab him.'

Deborah would, Olivia thought as she put down the phone and slowly made her way back to the kitchen, but with her looks she'd get away with it.

Seth said you were attractive.

Yes, but he was hardly likely to have told her she was plain. Not when she was his boss.

'How's your sister?'

'She's fine,' she replied, and watched his shirt tighten across his chest as he bent over to retrieve George's plastic chewing ring which had got itself wedged between the washing-machine and the tumble-drier.

Grab him, Deborah had said, and she would have done it if she'd been able to buy some new pyjamas, and she didn't look so white, and she'd been able to wash her hair.

No, you wouldn't, she thought as he straightened up and took the casserole out of the oven, because you're a wimp. A grade-A, three-star wimp.

Which was why, when dinner was over, she went meekly to her own bed and then lay awake for half the night, cursing her own timidity and feeling as frustrated as hell.

Jerry came round at midday on Sunday, clutching a casserole.

'I told Carol about what happened on Friday—the homeless man and the anti-retroviral drugs—and she insisted on me bringing this. I think she was worried you might starve to death.'

'Chance would be a fine thing, with Seth hovering around me like a broody hen,' she said, leading the way into the kitchen.

'Seth is still here?'

Jerry's surprise was obvious, and Olivia frowned slightly. 'Why shouldn't he still be here?'

'No reason.' Jerry put down the casserole. 'You look...' He paused, clearly searching for a tactful word, and settled for 'better'.

Hot and sexy would have been preferable, Olivia thought as she reached for the coffee-jar, but she supposed a girl had to settle for what compliments she could get. 'Would you like a coffee? Seth would have apoplexy if he knew I wasn't using the percolator, but I can't get the hang of it.'

'Instant's fine. Any word from the lab yet about your blood sample?'

'We heard yesterday that there's no sign of hepatitis C, but we're still waiting for the HIV. They did warn us it might take forty-eight hours so we're hoping to hear something at around five this afternoon.'

'I'd have thought they could have given you top priority,' Jerry grumbled, and she smiled as she spooned some coffee into a mug, then added water.

'You know what hospital bureaucracy is like. Everything's got to be done by the book.'

'Yes, but...' He flushed slightly as though he'd suddenly realised he might have been tactless. 'You're not worried about the result, are you? Statistically—'

'The odds are stacked pretty heavily against me being infected.' She nodded. 'I know. I wouldn't even have taken the test if Seth hadn't nagged and nagged and refused to take no for an answer. Milk and sugar?'

'Just black, please. I didn't know it was Seth who'd insisted,' Jerry said thoughtfully, taking the coffee from her outstretched hand. 'I did hear he caused a bit of a rumpus in the dispensary because they wanted to give you the shorter course of anti-retroviral drugs, and he insisted you have the full course.'

'Oh, he did, did he?' she said grimly. 'So I've got him to thank for all the hours I spent on the toilet. It's no joke, Jerry,' she continued as he laughed. 'I thought my entire stomach was being scoured out on Friday.'

'And Seth stayed with you?' Jerry shook his head. 'I think I've underestimated the man. Where is he?'

'In the sitting room, paint stripping the fireplace.'

Jerry choked over his coffee. 'Olivia, he doesn't know anything about paint stripping a fireplace.'

'I know he doesn't, but it seems to have become a matter of principle with him. His brawn against the vandals who painted it in the first place.' She frowned. 'Either that or he's taken to DIY in a big way.'

'Right.'

'He says he's down to the last coat of paint now, but I'm not holding my breath. He said the same thing at ten o'clock this morning.'

'Right,' Jerry said again. 'He's in the sitting room, you said?'

'Second door on the left,' she called after him as he made for the door. 'And tell him it's soup from a tin for lunch today whether he likes it or not.'

'Right,' Jerry said once more, and headed for the sitting room.

'It will look really lovely by the time I'm finished,' Seth said proudly as Jerry sat on the sofa and stared at the pink fireplace. 'It's Victorian cast iron, and you wouldn't believe the colours I've had to take off to get down to this last one.'

'Fascinating,' Jerry murmured. 'But what I'm more interested in is why you're still here. On Friday morning I distinctly remember you saying you were moving out.'

Seth threw down his paint scraper and sat back on his heels. 'What kind of jerk would walk out on a woman who might be HIV positive?'

'Seth, the likelihood of Olivia being HIV positive—'

'Is 0.2 to 0.5 per cent. I know. But while there's a chance—even the remotest of chances—I have to stay.'

Jerry took a sip of his coffee and gazed at Seth over the rim of his mug. 'So, after Olivia's got the all-clear from the lab, you're off?'

'Well, not immediately. Look, there's this fireplace to finish for a start, and she's bound to feel a bit shaky for a while,' Seth continued defensively, as a grin tugged at the corners of Jerry's lips. 'Those anti-retroviral drugs are murder on the system, so she'll need building up, and if I'm not here she'll go right back to eating those damn chill-cook foods.'

'So you've decided to become her minder after all, have you?'

'Only temporarily. Purely temporarily,' Seth insisted, and Jerry's smile widened.

'Right,' he said, and Seth glowered at him and went back to scraping the paint off the fireplace.

The last coat of paint finally came off at four o'clock and Seth took George out for a celebratory walk. At least, that's what he said he was doing but Olivia had a strong suspicion he was really hoping that Morrison's might be open on a Sunday so he could boast of his triumph.

Men were such big kids at times, she thought with a chuckle as she opened all the windows to try to get rid of the paint-stripper fumes, but at least his absence meant she had the house to herself for a while, which was good.

Except it was so quiet. So very quiet. Of course, she normally had George padding around after her, but it wasn't that, and she knew it wasn't.

She missed the sound of Seth's voice. She missed talking to him and laughing with him. She missed listening to his stories of his childhood on the Isle of Skye and hearing about all the crazy things he and his brothers had done when they'd been children. It wasn't just that he was an attractive sexy man, she missed *him*.

Which meant she was in big trouble because he'd leave when his ceiling was repaired and she'd be alone again with George.

'I can cope,' she told the microwave. 'I'm an independent career-woman now. It's what I wanted. To be independent, to be able to have affairs if I wanted, then walk away.' Except, of course, that when Seth walked away the only thing she'd have to look back on would be the sound of his laughter. And no career or life if the lab result wasn't good.

She glanced at the clock. Jerry was right. She should have heard something by now, which meant…

Nothing, she told herself firmly. The silence from the lab wasn't sinister or worrying—it just meant they were snowed under with work.

Seth clearly thought so, too, when he came back from his walk and didn't ask if anybody had phoned, but he was quick enough on his feet when the phone eventually did ring just before five o'clock, beating her into the hall by a mile.

'Ah,' he murmured as she hovered by his side, trying unsuccessfully to hear what the person at the other end of the phone was saying. 'Yes, but what about…?'

'What are they saying?' she hissed, and he flapped his hand at her to silence her.

Damnation, it should be her on the phone. It was her body, her future. Not that she was worried about the result or anything, but…

'Seth—'

'So, this means…?' He continued. 'I see. And there's no possibility of a mistake?'

Oh, get off the phone. Just get off the damn phone and tell me the worst, she thought as he nodded and murmured 'Ah' yet again.

'What did they say?' she said when he eventually replaced the receiver. 'Is it good news or…?'

He turned towards her, his face cracking into a wide, blinding smile. 'You're clear. There's no sign of HIV at all.'

Relief flooded through her. An overwhelming, shattering relief that made her want to laugh and cry at the same time.

'I *knew* I wouldn't be infected,' she exclaimed. 'I *knew* you were overreacting—making me take those awful horse pills. Jerry told me you insisted I have the full course, and there—you see—I didn't need them.'

'No, you didn't,' he murmured.

'I wasn't worried—of course I wasn't,' she continued. 'It was…it was just the inconvenience of having to take those pills and sign all those forms. And Deb,' she continued, her voice becoming shakier and shakier. 'She freaks out if she even cuts her finger, and I thought, How am I going to tell her? Not that I actually thought I was ever going to tell her because I *knew* I'd be all right—but that wretched diarrhoea seemed to go on and on, and I thought…I thought…'

'Liv, the test was negative,' he insisted, as tears began trickling down her cheeks. She tried to rub them away, but more just came.

'I don't know why I'm crying. It's stupid…so stupid…but I was so scared, Seth. I didn't know just how scared I was until you said…you said…'

She couldn't say any more. Couldn't get the words past the hard lump in her throat. Before she realised what was happening, he had reached for her and was holding her tight. So tight that she could feel his heart beating fast against her own. So tight that she could smell his warmth and feel the roughness of his shirt against her cheek, and she never ever wanted him to let go.

Grab him, Deb had said. *If you want him, just grab him.*

Dimly, she heard the microwave ping in the kitchen, and felt Seth's grasp around her beginning to loosen. All she had to say was, I want you. But where did you find the courage to say it? Men did it all the time, and they seemed to find it easy, or maybe they didn't. Maybe they found it hard, too, and would welcome it if you took the initiative.

'Seth…' She looked up at him, and his face was all dark planes and shadows in the hallway light. He looked hot, and dangerous, and every-thing she had always run away from in the past, but she wasn't running now. 'Seth, I...'

Say it, just say it, her heart whispered. But she couldn't, and he was stepping back from her, leaving her feeling cold, and empty, and stupid.

'Sounds like our dinner's ready,' he said.

Was it her imagination or did his voice sound odd, slightly constricted? He certainly didn't say much over dinner. She didn't say much either for fear she'd do something silly, like burst into tears all over again. It was a relief when it was half past ten and she could go to bed.

'Back to work tomorrow,' she said with a brightness she didn't feel when they stood to-gether outside her bedroom.

'You're sure you're fit enough to go back to work?' he asked as George raced past him to find his favourite spot at the end of her bed.

'Of course I'm fit enough. I'm not rushing to the loo any more, and now I know I don't have hepatitis C or HIV—well, life goes on, doesn't it?'

'Right.' He half turned to go, then stopped. 'If you should need me during the night—don't feel well—you know where I am.'

I need you now. 'Thanks, but I'm sure I'll sleep like a log.'

He nodded, and she held her breath, and he said goodnight, and she said goodnight, and she went into her bedroom and shut the door.

Twenty minutes later Seth lay stretched out on his bed, staring up at the ceiling.

He'd showed restraint. When she'd cried, and he'd held her in his arms, and had been all too devastatingly aware of how soft and warm she was, he'd showed restraint, and restraint was good. And frustrating and physically painful.

Maybe he ought to get up, try the cold-shower routine magazines were always advocating, except he'd probably meet Olivia in the hallway, and she'd undoubtedly be wearing those damn pyjamas again, and...

He turned over and thumped his pillows hard. Paint stripping. He would think about paint stripping. Lord, but he'd never realised what a job he'd taken on until he'd started. He'd had to peel off every single layer one by one. Strip off each coat little by little...

He let out a muttered oath, and hit his pillow again. Thinking about paint stripping was not helping. Thinking about stripping anything when Olivia was lying just a few feet away from him down the hall was a very bad idea.

Charlie. He would think about Charlie. Charlie had the right idea, partying every night, dating a different girl every week. That's what he'd do when he moved in with him. He'd dig out his little black book, phone up some of his old girlfriends and get himself back into circulation. Once he was back in circulation, everything would be fine.

Of course, he'd have to make sure he'd cooked enough casseroles to put in Olivia's freezer before he left, otherwise she'd go straight back to eating those chill-cook foods again and lose all the lovely curves he'd felt when he'd held her. The swell of her hips, the lush softness of her breasts...

'Oh, hell,' he groaned as he thumped his pillows yet again, and desperately—frantically—tried to think of something that wouldn't remind him of Olivia.

Olivia lay on her bed with George curled up beside her and stared at the ceiling. She was a wimp. There was no two ways about it, she was definitely a wimp.

What was she doing here with George when it was Seth she wanted? Seth rolling hard on top of her, Seth touching her and giving her everything she had ever wanted.

Then go to him.

But what if she crawled into his bed, and he turned round and said, I'd rather not, thank you very much? She'd die of shame and mortification.

But what if he didn't say, No, thank you very much? What if he smiled with that wonderful smile of his and reached for her and kissed her like last time, but this time he didn't stop? What if he pulled her close to him, and threaded his fingers through her hair, and whispered her name, and touched her all over, and then slid right into her?

'Oh, hell, George,' she whispered, and heard him snore in reply.

Are you a woman or a mouse? her mind whispered. *The whole point of you moving from Edinburgh to Glasgow was so you could become the new independent, in-your-face Olivia, so get out of that bed and go to him.*

But what if he looked shocked—what if he looked horrified—what if…?

The world ends tonight, and you never get this chance again?

And before she had even realised that she had made a conscious decision, she had got out of bed and was walking down the corridor.

CHAPTER EIGHT

'WHAT'S wrong, Liv?' Seth asked, switching on his bedside light and levering himself upright as she opened the door. 'Do you feel ill—need help?'

You'd better believe it, she thought, mesmerised by the sight of his broad, muscular shoulders and equally muscular chest glowing in the lamplight. *Because now I'm here, I don't know what to do.*

'Seth...I...I...'

Oh, hell, she didn't know what to say either, but she couldn't stand in the doorway all night, her mouth opening and closing like a floundering fish.

Actions speak louder than words. She'd read that somewhere, and doing something seemed slightly less stupid than simply staring at him so she walked slowly towards him and sat down on the edge of his bed.

'Liv...?'

His voice had deepened, roughened, but there was an edge of uncertainty to it, too, and it was that uncertainty which gave her the courage to reach out and hesitantly—oh, so hesitantly—touch his cheek.

His eyes closed briefly, then they flew open again, and before she could chicken out—before she could get cold feet and high-tail it straight back to her bedroom—she did the only thing she could think of. She leant forward and kissed him.

For a second he sat motionless, and a wave of embarrassment flooded through her. He didn't want her. He was going to say, Thanks, but, no, thanks. And she was going to be so mortified, and then he'd leave in the morning, and…

But he didn't say, Thanks, but, no, thanks. Suddenly he groaned against her lips, and before she could say anything or do anything he had pulled her down, rolled her under him and was kissing her back, and it was exactly as she had imagined, only better, much better.

'I thought you were going to tell me to go away,' she gasped as his lips teased and tasted hers, then tracked down her throat to plant a row of burning kisses along her collarbone.

'*Go away?*' he exclaimed, his fingers struggling to undo the buttons of her pyjama top. 'Why the hell would I tell you to go away when this is what I've been wanting to do ever since I moved in?'

'Then why didn't you say so?' she protested, shivering slightly as he parted her top, leaving her breasts bare. 'I've been wanting to jump on you for days, but I thought you'd be horrified—'

'Delighted—I'm delighted.' He chuckled huskily as his fingers cupped one of her breasts and his thumb teased the nipple until it hardened into a throbbing, aching point. 'Can't you tell how delighted I am?'

'I'm sorry about the pyjamas,' she said, tracing his throat with her lips as his free hand began to ease her trousers down. 'I meant to buy new ones—sexy ones...'

'Then buy another pair of these. Better still, buy ten pairs in case they become a discontinued line.'

'You think my pyjamas are sexy?' she said, only to arch up against him with a gasp when his lips closed around her nipple. 'Seth, I think you need help.'

'I just need you.' He laughed against her breast, making her shudder and squirm as tiny darts of desire shot through her.

And I need you, she thought.

Lord, but he felt so good against her. Heavier and more muscular than Phil had been, but less tentative. There was nothing tentative about Seth. Every touch of his fingers and his lips was sure and certain, every taste of his tongue was guaranteed to give her maximum pleasure, until simply touching him and being touched wasn't enough.

'Are you sure about this, Liv?' he said raggedly when his boxer shorts were gone and there was nothing between them but hot, fevered skin. 'Because if you're not…'

'It's a bit late to ask me that now, don't you think?' she gasped back breathlessly, wrapping her legs around him, biting him lightly on the shoulder, urging him on, wanting him inside her.

'And there was me thinking you were lavender and lace and home-made bread,' he groaned, his body rigid with tension as he rolled her on top of him.

'You thought I was what?' she said in confusion, writhing against him as he cupped her bottom to bring her closer to him.

'Home-made bread,' he repeated, rolling her back under him. 'I'm sushi, and you're home-made bread.'

'And you're crazy,' she said, beginning to laugh, only to cry out when he suddenly drove deep inside her, filling her with his hardness.

'Oh, yes—*yes*. Don't stop, please—please, don't stop.'

He didn't. As though her cry had broken something inside him, he began surging into her, and she surged, too, against him, with him, and the pressure began building and building, and she was half sobbing with need, and suddenly she was there, and she felt herself going right over the edge, falling and falling, her whole body convulsing and throbbing and exploding in his arms.

He reached the same heights a heartbeat behind her, and she heard his cry, felt the shudders running down his back as he jerked against her, and then he collapsed onto her chest with a groan, and she held him tight as the aftershocks consumed them.

'I didn't know,' she whispered into his hair when her heart rate eventually returned to normal. 'I didn't know it could ever be like this.'

'Neither did I,' he murmured. 'You're one very special lady, Olivia Mackenzie.'

'I'm special?' she faltered, and he lifted his head and grinned down at her.

'Liv, you are mind-blowing.'

He thought she was mind-blowing. Not dull and boring, but mind-blowing, and she sighed as he gently brought her round to him so she lay curled up against his chest.

'And now you need sleep,' he continued. 'You've been one very sick puppy for the last couple of days, and I should have gone slower just now, but I wanted you so badly, and—'

'Are you sorry for what we did?' she said uncertainly, and he planted a soft kiss on her forehead.

'Of course I'm not sorry, but you've been ill, and what you need most now is sleep. If you're going back to work tomorrow—'

'We both have to go back to work tomorrow,' she said sleepily. 'It's not fair to leave Jerry and Tony holding the fort alone.'

'I guess not.' He yawned, wrapping his other arm around her to bring her closer, and as he felt asleep with his head resting on the top of her shoulder, all she could think was, *I never knew. I never knew it could be like this.*

Seth sighed as he gazed up at the sunlight streaming through the window. He was alone in bed, but even if the space beside him hadn't still been warm he knew he couldn't possibly have dreamt what had happened last night. Which meant he was in big trouble.

He'd done his level best to keep his hands off her, but he'd failed, and now the best thing he could do—the only thing—would be to pack his bag and go. It was what he'd always done in the past. A smile to the woman in question, a couple of throw-away lines which could mean anything and always meant nothing, and then he'd walked away as fast as he could.

Except that Liv wasn't just the woman in question, he realised as he heard her call to George, and the big dog padded along the hall and, instead of going downstairs, came straight into his bedroom. She was Liv.

Liv who smiled at him over the breakfast table. Liv who laughed with him, and argued with him. Liv who had taken on this big old house and George, because she said she needed something and someone who needed her.

'She's something special, George,' he murmured when the dog clambered up onto the bed beside him. 'Special, and different, and unique.'

George pricked up his ears quizzically, and Seth shook his head. 'No, it isn't just the sex. It's…' He struggled to find the right words. 'It's more than sex. I want to take care of her, to keep her safe. If anything should ever happen to her…'

His heart twisted inside him at the thought of a world without Liv. It would be so empty, so dark, so grey. For years he'd run away from relationships, never wanting to get too close, never wanting to give too much of himself to anyone, but now…

'I need her, George,' he said as the dog rolled over onto his back with his paws in the air. 'I don't know why I do—or how it's happened—but I need her. She's so different to anyone I've ever met before. She's loving, and gentle, and infuriating, and I *need* her. I don't want to walk away. I want to stay with her for the rest of my life, making her happy.'

George gave a short, sharp bark, and Seth laughed softly.

'Yes, I know. I don't understand it either, unless…' He sat up so quickly that George had to scrabble to hold onto the bed covers. 'I've fallen in love with her, haven't I, George? This is what falling in love means. Wanting to be with the person you love all the time. Wanting to hold onto them and take care of them, and just be there for them through the good times and the bad.'

George didn't look certain, and Seth couldn't blame him. Up until now he'd never believed such an emotion existed either, but up until now he'd never met a woman like Olivia. What he felt for her was what he'd never felt for anybody else, and he couldn't let her go, he couldn't let her slip through his fingers.

'George, I'm going to ask your mother to marry me. Yes, I know I said marriage was for the brain dead,' he continued as the dog stared at him, 'but you know something? I don't care. I don't care if being married to Liv gives me the appearance of a man who's had a full frontal lobotomy. I love her, and I want to marry her.'

And as George let out another bark, Seth laughed, threw back the covers and got out of bed to go downstairs and tell Olivia.

'Have you seen George?' she said as he went into the kitchen and found her standing by the stove. 'I called to him, but—'

'He's curled up on my bed.'

She sighed, and turned back to the pot she was stirring. 'I should have shut the door properly. If he gets even the sniff of a warm bed he's straight in it.'

'Can't say I blame him,' he said, walking up to her and wrapping his arms around her. 'I'd be just the same if the bed in question had you in it. You OK this morning?'

She turned so he could kiss her. 'Couldn't be better. How about you?'

'Fantastic. In fact, I'd like to do this every morning.'

'Oh, I think that could be arranged,' she said, licking into his mouth and smiling when she felt him shudder. 'Except we'll only be able to do it when you stay here. George doesn't like change so I can't see me ever being able to stay over at your place once your ceiling's fixed.'

'That isn't what I meant,' he murmured. 'What I meant is I'd like to move in here permanently. What I really meant is, I want us to get married.'

For a second she thought he was joking, but one look at his smiling face told her he wasn't, and an icy chill of dismay ran down her back.

Married?

She'd only been divorced for six months. She was just beginning to enjoy her freedom and independence, and he wanted her to give them both up and *get married?*

'Have you been at the cooking sherry this morning?' she said, striving to sound light, casual, and the smile on his face wavered.

'Isn't this the moment when you're supposed to flutter your eyelashes and say, ''Oh, Seth, but this is so sudden, you've taken me by surprise but, yes, I'll marry you?'''

She tried to smile, and failed miserably. 'Seth, I like having you here—'

'That's good—positive.'

'And you can stay for as long as you want—'

'Permanence—that sounds good, too. So...'

'But I don't want to marry you. I left Edinburgh and Phil because I wanted to be an independent career-woman.'

He loosened his hold on her. 'Liv, you left Phil because he was playing around.'

Just as you might—probably will. 'Seth, if you like being here so much, why can't we just live together? Lots of people do.'

'I'm not lots of people,' he said stubbornly. 'I want us to get married so you can't ever run away.'

'You might want to one day.'

'I won't.'

She stared up into his handsome face, and her heart sank. He looked so sure, so certain, but how could she make him understand that the thought of marrying again made her feel quite ill? She'd been convinced she'd been doing the right thing when she'd married Phil, but she hadn't even used up all the sheets and towels they'd been given as wedding presents when her marriage had been over, and to go through that all again…'

'Seth…'

He wasn't listening. His eyes had slid to the pan on the stove, and he was frowning.

'What *is* that mess you're cooking?'

'Scrambled eggs.'

'Liv, that is not scrambled eggs. That is battered, mashed and thoroughly killed eggs. Give me the pan, and let me do it.'

She watched him dump her eggs into the bin, and when he took a fresh pan out of the cupboard she tried again.

'Seth, you do understand, don't you? You can stay with me for as long as you want, but I'm not marrying you.'

He threw her a super-confident, completely certain grin. 'Not today perhaps, or tomorrow, but I'll talk you round.'

And as he picked up the whisk and began beating the eggs, she wondered what she would have to say to convince him that she'd meant what she'd said, and she was never going to change her mind, ever.

'It is so good to see you back.' Babs beamed as Olivia joined her at the top of the examination room. 'How do you feel? I have to say you're still looking a bit peaky.'

'I'm fine—honestly.' Olivia smiled. 'Any problems over the weekend?'

Babs opened her mouth, then closed it again. 'Nothing we couldn't handle.'

Which meant there'd been a problem—a big one.

'OK, spit it out,' Olivia sighed. 'What disaster occurred over the weekend?'

Babs glanced down the examination room to where Seth had just joined Jerry outside cubicle 3, and shook her head. 'Could we talk about this in private?'

Curiouser and curiouser, and distinctly worrying.

'It will have to be some time this afternoon—preferably after we've finished our shift,' Olivia declared. 'The waiting room's full, and I've a meeting with Admin at lunchtime, plus masses of paperwork to catch up on.'

'This afternoon will be fine,' Babs said, and as the sister hurried away, a faint frown creased Olivia's forehead.

Babs was normally completely unflappable, but she was definitely in a flap this morning. In a flap and worried. Jerry hadn't seemed worried. He'd hailed her with a bright smile when she'd arrived, made a joke about doctors having to take a dose of their own medicine, then had got on with his work as usual. But Babs was not a happy woman.

'Eight-year-old with breathing difficulties, Olivia,' Fiona declared, breaking into her thoughts. 'Asthmatic since he was four. His GP sent him in because his pulse is 140 per minute, and he has a peak expiratory flow of 50 per cent.'

'Where is he?'

'Cubicle 6. His mother's with him, and I don't know who's more uptight—the boy or his mother.'

Which meant that whatever Babs's problem was, it would have to wait until later, Olivia thought as she followed Fiona into the cubicle.

'Seth, you look like the cat that got the cream this morning,' Jerry observed, stepping back to allow Fiona to wheel the last patient he'd seen off to X-Ray.

'I feel like the cat.' Seth grinned, and the specialist registrar's eyebrows rose.

'Do I take it things have moved beyond first base with you and Olivia?'

'Way beyond first base, Jerry. In fact, I've asked her to marry me.'

'You asked her to…?' The specialist registrar's mouth fell open. 'Seth, I'm delighted for you both—honestly I am—but isn't this a bit sudden? I mean, you only met her three weeks ago.'

'Like all the books say, sometimes it needs just one look to know you've met the woman you want to spend the rest of your life with.'

Jerry's mouth dropped even further. 'So…so when's the wedding?'

'Well, she hasn't actually said yes,' Seth admitted. 'In fact, she said no. I think she probably feels as you do—that I should have waited a little longer before I asked her—but I'll talk her round.'

'Right.' Jerry nodded, still looking slightly pole-axed. 'But you really did ask her to marry you?'

Seth frowned at him. 'Jerry, people get married all the time. They settle down, have kids. What's so surprising about that?'

For a second Jerry said nothing, then he threw back his head and laughed. 'Nothing, Seth. Absolutely nothing at all.'

'Mrs Johnstone, your son really must have his bronchodilator with him all the time,' Olivia said as she led the very relieved mother out of cubicle 6. 'I know it can be hard with children—they don't want to be seen as different to their friends—but the bronchodilator is the only way he's going to keep attacks like this at bay. Do you have a peak-flow meter at home so you can monitor Sam's asthma?'

'He hates me using it,' Mrs Johnstone sighed, 'but I'm going to accept no arguments from him from now on. I don't want another day like today, if I can avoid it.'

Olivia pulled a piece of paper from her pocket and wrote down a telephone number. 'The hospital has a self-help group for children with asthma. It's very informal—just a few parents and their children getting together once a week-but perhaps if Sam met other children who have asthma...?'

'He might realise he's not the only one.' Mrs Johnstone nodded and took the piece of paper Olivia was holding out to her. 'Thanks, Doctor. I'll certainly phone them.' She turned to her son as Fiona ushered him out of the cubicle. 'And as for you, young man—you're going to carry that bronchodilator from now on if I have to tie it round your neck with a bit of string.'

'Mother love.' Fiona chuckled as Mrs Johnstone and Sam walked out of the examination room together, and Olivia laughed.

'I'd probably be the same if it was me.'

Not that she was planning on having children any time soon, and neither was she going to get married again, no matter what Seth said.

Why couldn't he leave things the way they were? she wondered irritably as she saw Babs beckoning to him from outside cubicle 1. Last night had been incredible, and she was more than happy to have more of the same—*you betcha,* her body replied enthusiastically—but *married?* No way. Somehow she had to talk him out of his crazy idea but, judging by how persistent he'd been with her fireplace, it wasn't going to be easy.

'Oh, hell, it looks like we've got an overdose in cubicle 1,' Fiona groaned as they watched Babs rush out of the cubicle and return equally quickly with the stomach pump. 'I hate ODs.'

So did Olivia. They were messy and difficult to perform, and the patients fought you all the way.

'I suppose I'd better ask Babs and Seth if they want any help,' Fiona continued reluctantly, but she was back at Olivia's side in seconds, her face tight. 'It's Mary Miller, Olivia, and Seth says it looks bad.'

It did.

'Do we know what kind of pills she took?' Olivia asked as Seth gently began to ease the lubricated tube of the stomach pump down Mary's throat. The woman gagged and retched and, despite being drowsy, still tried to fight against it.

'Paracetamol washed down with vodka, according to the empty bottle her neighbour found,' Seth said grimly.

Paracetamol. Known to every A and E department in the country as the housewives' overdose drug of choice because women thought it would help them to slip swiftly and painlessly away, whereas the reality was that they all too often lived on, crippled with acute liver damage.

'How many?' Olivia said, reaching out to restrain Mary's legs as she began to writhe and kick in earnest.

'Sixty, given the number of empty packs there were, but…'

Olivia nodded. The government had imposed a crackdown on the sale of paracetamol, limiting the amount that any individual could buy, but there was nothing to stop a determined woman—or man—from visiting every chemist in their area.

'You said her neighbour found her,' Olivia said. 'Do we know when she took the pills?'

Seth shook his head. 'Her neighbour dropped in for a coffee just before eleven and found her flat out on the sofa. She remembers seeing her returning home after taking her kids to school at around nine, so if she took the pills then…'

The pills would already have left her stomach, Olivia finished for him mentally, and be on their way through her intestines, causing maximum damage to her liver.

'Why did she do it, Olivia?' Seth continued, his voice harsh, bitter as he added charcoal to the lubricated tube. 'Why now? I could understand her doing it if Alec had been hitting her again, but there's no fresh injuries on her face, so why now, just after she'd taken her kids to school?'

'I guess everybody has their own breaking point,' Olivia murmured. 'Maybe it was something small, something you and I would have considered trivial in the light of everything else she's had to endure, but it was enough for her to decide she just didn't want to go on living any more.'

'I wish her husband could see this,' Seth exclaimed, his eyes dark with anger. 'I wish I could make him watch while we do this, and somehow feel Mary's pain. Why is it the innocent who always suffer, Olivia—*why?*'

'I don't know,' she said sadly. 'I wish I did, but I don't.'

Eventually the liquid coming through the stomach pump began to run clear. The charcoal Seth had inserted into the tube would have absorbed any paracetamol that had been left lingering in Mary's stomach, but they wouldn't know for three days whether they'd extracted all the paracetamol or whether some of it—or indeed all of it—had travelled into her intestines.

'What a mess, Liv,' Seth sighed when Mary was finally transferred to Intensive Care. 'What a bloody awful mess.'

'She might be lucky,' Olivia said gently. 'We could have got all the paracetamol out.'

'And if we haven't, she'll have liver damage. She's thirty-four years old, Liv, with three kids under the age of eight and a husband who beats the living daylights out of her when he's drunk. What kind of life is that?'

'Maybe—if she survives—this will persuade her to leave her husband?' she said hesitantly, and Seth's lips twisted.

'I'd like to think it would, but you know something? I wouldn't bet on it.'

Neither would Olivia.

*   *   *

It was a long day. Long, and tiring, and frustrating, and Olivia's meeting with Admin was a disaster. They weren't happy with her unit-throughput figures and she lost her temper, which was completely unlike her, and by the time the meeting was over the atmosphere could have been cut with a knife.

'Sometimes I wonder why I ever took this job,' she told the mound of paperwork on her desk. 'I must have been out of my mind.'

She was doubly convinced of her own insanity when Babs arrived at her office door at five o'clock, looking tense and unhappy.

'Look, Babs, will you just spit it out?' she said after the sister had made three false starts, and she was still none the wiser as to what had happened at the weekend. 'Whatever it is can't be that bad.'

'Somebody's taking drugs from our store cupboard. Amphetamines.'

She'd been wrong. It could be that bad. 'Taking?' she repeated. 'You mean stealing?'

Babs nodded. 'It was quiet on Sunday so I decided to take a quick inventory, and our stock's far too low. Whoever is stealing them isn't taking enough to be a supplier, but they're taking enough to suggest they have a serious habit.'

'But the store cupboard is always kept locked,' Olivia protested. 'The only members of staff who have authorised access are you, me, Jerry, Tony and Seth.'

'Exactly.'

Olivia stared at Babs in dismay. The sister was saying that one of them was addicted to amphetamines, but surely it couldn't be one of them—could it?

'Perhaps one of us forgot to lock the door,' she exclaimed, desperately clutching at straws. 'It can happen—a moment's forgetfulness, a second's distraction—and somebody was passing—'

'Olivia, this must have been going on for weeks, and I think we would have noticed a stranger constantly passing through the trauma room.'

She was right. They would have.

'Babs—'

'I didn't take the amphetamines, and I'd stake my reputation that you didn't, which means...'

It had to be Seth, Jerry or Tony.

Not Seth. It couldn't be Seth. He'd never be so stupid, and neither would Jerry. But would Tony?

Olivia straightened up in her seat. 'Could you ask Seth and Jerry to come to my office, please, Babs?'

The sister hurried out of the office, relief plain on her face that the problem was no longer hers, and Olivia put her fingers to her forehead to try to ease the tension headache she could already feel beginning to form there.

Lord, but this was turning out to be a really lousy day. She should have taken a sickie. If she'd listened to Seth and taken a sickie, she could have been at home in bed now instead of facing the unpalatable fact that a member of A and E was stealing uppers.

'Well, my money's on young Tony being the culprit,' Seth declared after he and Jerry had listened to her revelations.

'Oh, come on, Seth, that's hardly fair,' Olivia protested. 'I know you've never particularly liked him, but whatever happened to innocent until proven guilty?'

'He's too full of bounce—too constantly high.'

'Because he's young,' she exclaimed. 'When you're young you have more energy—'

'And his mind wanders,' Seth continued, as though she hadn't spoken. 'Remember that woman with malaria, and Mrs Macmillan's ''do not resuscitate'' form?'

'Seth, those were mistakes. We've all made mistakes, but that doesn't mean we're all popping amphetamines. Jerry, what do you think?'

The specialist registrar frowned as he sat back in his seat. 'I think we need a lot more than mere suspicion to accuse him of something as big as this.'

'Well, I don't,' Seth retorted. 'I think we should simply ask him outright whether he's stealing from the store cupboard.'

'Oh, brilliant,' Olivia said, shooting him a withering glance. 'And if he says no, we've accused him without any proof, and we could end up in all kinds of trouble.'

'And if he says no, and he's actually *guilty,* we're not going to be any further forward,' Jerry chipped in, but Seth wasn't placated.

'So how are we going to get this proof?' he demanded. 'Hang about the store cupboard for the foreseeable future in the hope that he—or somebody else—will go in and come out again with their pockets stuffed with uppers?'

Phil used to do that, she remembered as she stared across at Seth's irate face—use sarcasm to make her feel foolish and inadequate—and she was damned if she was going to put up with it again.

'That's exactly what we're going to do,' she said acidly. 'This whole sorry affair has to be handled with tact—'

'To hell with tact,' Seth protested, and Jerry looked from him to Olivia with clear concern.

'I think we're all getting a little bit over-heated here,' he said in his best let's-all-calm-down voice, but Seth wasn't listening.

'If you're too soft to ask Tony, *I'll* ask him.'

'No, I am *not* too soft,' Olivia retorted, 'but neither do I lose my head when I'm not winning an argument.'

Seth's eyebrows snapped down. 'You're saying I do?'

'Let's just say I think you could do with some anger management courses,' she retorted.

'Olivia—Seth,' Jerry protested, but they both ignored him.

'At least my solution is to *do* something, rather than just sitting around waiting for something to happen,' Seth flared.

'Your solution is to go in all guns blazing without thinking of the consequences,' she threw back at him. 'Tony could sue us for slander—'

'Oh, for crying out loud,' he exclaimed. 'I don't see how asking somebody a straight question can mean we'll end up being accused of slander.'

'Well, I can. Which is probably why I'm the boss and you're not,' she snapped back before she could stop herself. She heard Jerry groan.

A dark shade of livid colour swept across Seth's cheeks and she bit her lip. She hadn't meant to say that—to use her position to end an argument—but what he was suggesting was not only ridiculous but potentially catastrophic.

'Seth, listen—'

'Why?' he said grimly. 'After all—as you've just made all too abundantly clear—you're the boss, and you know everything. In fact, I'm surprised you even bothered to ask me to sit in on this meeting when you clearly think so little of my opinion.'

'And now you're being childish,' she protested. 'You know perfectly well that I couldn't run this department without you.'

'So I'm good enough to be your general dogsbody, but not good enough to be allowed a voice, is that it?' he demanded, and neither of them noticed Jerry tiptoeing quietly out of the room. 'Is this how you used to talk to Phil? If it is, I'm not surprised he walked.'

She gazed across at him, her mouth working soundlessly for a second, and when she spoke her voice was uneven, shaky. 'That's a horrible thing to say. You know nothing about my marriage—nothing at all.'

'Liv, I'm sor—'

'What do you know about my marriage—about anybody's marriage?' she continued, so angry now that she didn't notice the contrition in his face. 'You've never been married. In fact, you've spent your entire life running away from any kind of commitment.'

'Liv—'

'All that nonsense you said this morning about us getting married... Ye gods, your idea of long-term commitment is a long weekend.'

A blaze of anger darkened his blue eyes. 'If that's what you think of me, I'm surprised you bother with me at all.'

'I'm beginning to wonder the same thing myself,' she said, her voice a good deal harder than his. 'In fact, I think it might be better if you found somewhere else to live until your ceiling's fixed.'

He met her gaze for a second, then got his feet. 'Fine. I'll be out of your place before you get home tonight.'

He'd be out of her house before she got home? She stared at him aghast as he walked towards the door. What had she done? She didn't want him to leave—she'd never intended telling him to leave. The words had just slipped out because she'd been so angry, and he'd suddenly reminded her so much of Phil. But he wasn't Phil, and she didn't want him to go.

'Seth...' He turned to face her, his face harder than she'd ever seen it, and a hard lump began to form in her throat, a lump that seemed to grow and grow. She swallowed hard to try to get rid of it, but it wouldn't go away. She wasn't going to beg. If he was just going to walk away without even attempting to make her change her mind, she wasn't going to beg.

'Will...will you be all right?' she managed to say. 'I mean, have you got somewhere to stay?'

'Charlie has a spare room.'

His voice was cold, implacable, and the lump in her throat got bigger. 'Oh. I see. Seth—'

It was too late. He'd gone.

Well, you've done it now, she thought as she listened to the sound of his footsteps growing fainter and fainter in the corridor outside. *You've well and truly done it now.*

It was for the best, she told herself as she gazed down at her hands and saw they were shaking. She and Seth... It would never have worked. Eventually he would have got bored with her, and as for his crazy idea of them getting married... He wasn't the marrying kind, despite all his protestations, and she wanted independence.

And you've got it, she realised as she sat in her office and heard nothing but the ticking of the clock on her desk. Well, she was a big girl now, and she'd survive. Relationships ended all the time. This was just part of the learning curve of her new life of independence.

'I'm fine. Really, I am,' she told the empty room. 'I'm the new independent, in-your-face Olivia, so I'm fine.'

And as a tear trickled slowly down her cheek and splashed onto the desk in front of her, she knew she would be fine eventually. It would just take time, and time was the one thing she had plenty of.

CHAPTER NINE

'THIS is the life, Seth, isn't it?' Charlie beamed as he admired his reflection in the mirror over the kitchen sink. 'Two guys sharing a place, enjoying themselves, answerable to nobody.'

'Oh, yes, this is certainly the life,' Seth answered without enthusiasm.

'So are you out on the pull tonight, looking for a bit of the old between-the-sheets entertainment?' Charlie asked, slipping his comb in the inside pocket of his jacket and dumping his cereal bowl into the sink beside the other dirty dishes from the night before.

'I thought I might have a quiet night in.'

'*Again?* Seth, my old buddy, my old pal, you moved in with me three days ago, and you haven't been out on a date once. Look, why don't I give Mandy a ring, ask if she's got a friend?'

'Thanks, but no thanks,' Seth said hurriedly, and Charlie shrugged.

'Your choice, but you're missing out on a whole lot of fun.' He made for the door. 'I'll be late back tonight, but don't wait up for me. And

if you hear a lot of noise coming from my bedroom...' He smirked. 'Just ignore it.'

I wish I could ignore you, Seth thought with
feeling as Charlie slammed the front door on his
way out.

Why in the world had he ever moved in with
him? He must have been mad.

No, not mad. Angry. Angry with Olivia.

Angry because she'd reminded him that she'd
got the clinical director's post and he hadn't. So
angry that he'd lashed out at her, saying awful
things, dreadful things, things which could
never be taken back.

'Seth, how could you have been so dumb?'
Jerry had exclaimed in disbelief when he'd told
him what had happened.

He wondered the same thing as he stared morosely at the dishes Charlie had left in the sink,
then walked out of the kitchen and deliberately
shut the door.

So Olivia was his boss—so what? Only a
very insecure man would have let that bother
him. Only a *really* insecure man would have let
it bother him to the extent that he'd lash out at
her the way he had.

He had been so *stupid.* He was good at his
job, and she was good at hers. He could never
have coped with the pen-pushers in Admin the

way she did, or have her patience to tackle the mounds of paperwork. He was a hands-on doctor. That was where he shone, and Olivia shone at organising, and coaxing, and fixing things. It didn't make him lesser, just different.

Which meant that somehow he had to undo the damage he'd done through those uncalled-for remarks about Phil. He could start by apologising for his childishness. Then he could ask her out to dinner, and over dinner he could switch on the old Hardcastle charm, and she...

She'd tell him that she didn't want him back because she didn't want to marry him.

So much for plan A. Hell, he should never have asked her to marry him quite so quickly—he could see that now. Good grief, she'd only been divorced for six months so she was bound to be wary, unwilling to commit. He should have bided his time, waited until she realised that she needed him as much as he needed her. But he hadn't and now he was going to have to re-group and start again more slowly.

Except that he didn't want to go slowly. He wanted her back now. It could take him weeks—months—to breach her defences, and he didn't want to wait weeks or months. He loved her, and he wanted to marry her—plus he had a horrible suspicion that if he didn't get out of Charlie's place soon, he was going to kill him.

Somehow he had to ingratiate himself back into Olivia's good books. If he could only do that and get himself back into her house, he just knew he could make everything all right. If all she initially wanted him back for was as a lover, he could live with that. If she would only take him back as a paying lodger, he could live with that, too. He just wanted to be close to her, to be near her, to watch over her and keep her safe, but how?

'Seth looks to be in a better mood today,' Jerry observed as he saw the consultant smile at one of the junior nurses on his way across the examination room.

'Good,' Olivia replied.

'It makes everything so much easier when we all get along, doesn't it?' the specialist registrar continued gamely. 'I mean, life's too short to harbour petty grudges or brood on imaginary wrongs, don't you think?'

'I couldn't agree more,' Olivia agreed, and Jerry gave up on subtlety.

'Olivia, won't you just forgive him and take him back?'

'There's nothing to forgive,' she protested. 'OK, so maybe he said some hurtful things, but I did, too. I'm not angry with him—at least, not any more.'

'Then how come he's living with Charlie, and you're on your own again?' the specialist registrar said bluntly.

'It was all...' She coloured slightly. 'It was all getting a bit heavy.'

'You mean because he asked you to marry him?'

The colour on her cheeks darkened to crimson. 'He told you that?'

'Olivia, Seth and I have been friends ever since I started work here, and he was so happy, so over the moon when he told me that he'd asked you to marry him—of course he told me.'

'Then he'll also have told you that I said no,' Olivia said awkwardly, and Jerry nodded.

'Look, it's none of my business why you said no, but I do know that though Seth can be a prize idiot at times—taking the hump because you said you were the boss is a prime example—he's a good bloke, a decent bloke.'

'Taking the hump is why he walked, Jerry.'

'My understanding is you told him to go,' Jerry said gently, and the colour on her cheeks darkened even more. 'Olivia, Seth's too big a man to let something as unimportant as you being his boss bother him.'

'Jerry, it really doesn't matter now how the row started,' she murmured. 'The bottom line is that he and I... We don't want the same things, so it's best we split up now and prevent a lot of heartache.'

'And has it?' the specialist registrar pressed. 'Prevented a lot of heartache?'

'Jerry—'

'The very man I'm looking for.' Babs beamed. 'We've a young woman in cubicle 4 who can't get her contact lenses out. She only started wearing them three weeks ago, and she's in a dreadful panic—convinced they're going to be permanently stuck to her eyeballs.'

'Have you tried saline drops, and then pinching them out between your thumb and finger?' the specialist registrar asked, and Babs gave him a round-eyed-what-an-amazing-suggestion look.

'Duh, and there was me thinking I could simply yank them out with a scalpel. Of course I've tried saline drops and my fingers, but every time I get anywhere near her she starts blinking and flinching, and I thought maybe your manifold masculine charms might calm her down.'

'Babs, after flattery like that, you can have anything you want.' Jerry grinned. 'What's she like—tall, blonde, pneumatic?'

'She is, actually,' the sister said with a chuckle, 'so I suggest you keep reminding yourself that you're married when you examine her.'

Jerry laughed, and Olivia tried to join in, but her laughter sounded false even to her own ears. Jerry meant well—she knew he did—but he didn't understand any more than Seth did.

If she couldn't make a success of a relationship with a man like Phil, she didn't have a hope in hell of making a success of a relationship with a man like Seth. Maybe she could apologise for what she'd said, and he might apologise for what *he'd* said, but if they got back together again they'd only be postponing the inevitable. He may have thought she was exciting when they'd made love, but his excitement wouldn't last. Eventually he'd get bored and walk away, so it was better this way. Much better.

She just wished she could make George understand that. Ever since Seth had left he'd been rushing to the door whenever the doorbell rang, only to pad disconsolately back when he discovered it was only the postman or the delivery man, and this morning she'd actually found him curled up on Seth's bed.

'He was never going to stay with us permanently, George,' she'd said when she'd coaxed
him off the bed. 'You know it was simply a
temporary arrangement.'

George hadn't looked convinced. Her sister
Deborah had been even less convinced when
she'd telephoned to ask how things were going.

'What do you mean, he's moved out?'
Deborah had demanded. 'I thought he was staying with you until his ceiling was fixed?'

'He decided it would be more convenient if
he stayed in a flat nearer the hospital.'

'Yeah, right, Liv, and this is your big sister
you're talking to. What happened?'

*We made love, and he asked me to marry him,
and I said no, and then we had a row and I
asked him to leave.*

'Nothing happened, Deb.'

'So how come you're breaking your heart?'

'I'm not breaking my heart,' she'd protested.
'If I sound snuffly, it's only because I have a
slight head cold.'

'Liv—'

'I don't want to talk about it,' she'd said, and
had quickly put down the phone before the tears
she seemed to have such difficulty in suppress-
ing whenever she thought about Seth confirmed
her sister's worst suspicions.

She was not breaking her heart, she told herself as she walked slowly down the treatment room. She was just a little upset because of all the great sex she was missing. Independent career-women were allowed to be upset when a relationship ended. Independent career-women weren't machines, they were people, but she was *not* breaking her heart.

But she was just about to eat some very humble pie, she thought as she went out into the corridor, and came to a dead halt as she saw Tony Melville emerging from their dispensary. The junior doctor was putting something into his pocket, and as he looked up and saw her, she knew. He didn't have to say anything, she didn't have to say anything, she just knew. Seth had been right all along, and now it was up to her to deal with it.

'My office,' she said curtly, and he followed her without a word, but when he sat down across the desk from her, she couldn't restrain herself. 'Why, Tony? In God's name, *why?*'

'Because they're the only things that keep me awake,' he said simply.

She shook her head. 'Tony, I know a junior doctor's life is rough—the hours you have to work, being constantly at the beck and call of your superiors—but popping amphetamines...

You're a doctor, for God's sake. You of all people should know the damage they can do—what dependency on them can lead to.'

'I know—and you're right, but...'

'Has it all got too much for you?' she said gently as he came to a halt. 'Is that why you've been taking the pills?'

'*Too much for me?*' He let out a harsh, bitter laugh. 'Of course it's all too damned much for me. Do you know what it's like to be tired, Dr Mackenzie?'

'Yes, I do. In fact—'

'I don't mean the kind of tired in the way the general public would understand,' he continued as though she hadn't spoken. 'I mean tired to the bone. So tired I can hardly stand up some days.'

'Tony, you should have spoken to me, or to Seth, or to—'

'And said what?' he demanded. 'That I was tired? You would all have nodded and said, yes, it's rough, but we've all been there, done it, and it's just something you'll have to get through.'

'No, we wouldn't—'

'I hate this job, Dr Mackenzie. I hate the elderly patients we see who are walking social and medical disasters. I hate knowing that there's nothing we can do for them but send them upstairs to the geriatric ward, to our Gomer Hotel. Gomer. Standing for Get Out of My Emergency Room. An unloved geriatric patient on his or her last legs for no apparent reason.'

'Tony—'

'And the children. I hate seeing all the hurt children, the abused children and the dying children, because the only way I can cope with seeing them is to make myself feel nothing. To have no compassion, no sympathy. Because if I do, I'll go under.'

He was wrong, Olivia thought as she stared at him. Yes, they had to distance themselves slightly from the horrors they all too often saw, but if you allowed yourself to feel nothing for your patients, didn't care for them in their distress, you weren't a doctor any more. You'd become a machine.

She cleared her throat. 'Tony…'

His eyes met hers. 'This is the end of my career, isn't it?'

'I don't know what will happen,' she lied. 'I'll make out a report for Admin, and you'll be suspended from duty until they decide what action they want to take.'

'They'll bounce me, and I know I could make a good doctor. Not a doctor in A and E—I know

I can't cope with that—but perhaps as a GP in a quiet rural backwater.'

'Tony—'

'I'll stop taking the pills.' His eyes were fixed on her now, desperate, pleading. 'If I stop taking the pills, and you say nothing—let me finish my pre-registration year—I could make it worth your while. My parents have money—'

'Tony, don't make a bad situation even worse,' she said quickly. 'I have to fill in a report—you know I do—and now I want you to go home and stay there. You can tell Fiona and the others anything you like—'

'They'll know. They'll know I've been bounced.'

They would, too, because even if she only told Jerry, and Seth, it would get out. In a hospital it somehow always did.

'I'm sorry, Tony, but I'm afraid it's something you're just going to have to live with,' she said sadly.

'You never did like him, did you?' Olivia said to Seth when she told him about what had happened. 'Did you suspect right from the start that he was taking uppers?'

'Good lord, no,' he exclaimed. 'If I'd suspected anything like that, I would have told you immediately. I don't know why I didn't like him. It was nothing specific, just a niggling feeling that something wasn't quite right. And then when Babs said amphetamines were missing from our store cupboard...'

'You knew it was him.' Olivia sighed. 'I should have known it, too, shouldn't I? Recognised the warning signs.'

'How?' Seth protested. 'You said yourself that when you're young you have a lot more energy, so don't go beating yourself over the head with this.'

'I have to say I felt a bit sorry for him,' she said as they walked together down the corridor. 'I know I shouldn't,' she continued as his eyebrows rose, 'but it's rough when you're a junior doctor, all the jibes you have to take about being the thickest looking after the sickest.'

'You're too soft for your own good.'

He'd said that before, she remembered, just as she also remembered what had happened afterwards.

'Admin aren't happy with me either,' she said quickly, in case he remembered, too. 'Not only are my unit-throughput figures too low—'

'Your what?'

'It's the number of people we see and treat every hour,' she explained as he gazed at her, puzzled. 'We don't treat people any more, you see, we treat units.'

'Heaven save me from pen-pushers and their jargon,' he sighed, and she nodded.

'Well, not only are they not happy with my unit-throughput figures, they are now not happy with—how did they phrase it when I spoke to them about Tony at lunchtime? Ah, yes. ''You should have been aware that there was a problem in your department, Dr Mackenzie. That's what we're paying you for.'' '

'And just how are you supposed to know who's clean and who's not, unless you demand urine samples from us all every morning?' he demanded, and she sighed.

'That's what I said, but the bottom line is I'm the boss, so I carry the can.'

Damn, but she'd gone and used the 'B' word. The word which was like a red rag to a bull as far as he was concerned, and he was clearly thinking the same if the faint tinge of colour on his cheeks was anything to go by.

'I'd better let you go,' she said hurriedly. 'It's after five, and you must be eager to get home.'

He hasn't got a home, you idiot, she thought, groaning inwardly as she realised what she'd just said. He was staying with Charlie from

Dietetics, and she'd just gone and put her foot in it again.

She took a quick step forward, meaning to beat a hasty retreat into her office, only to see him bar her way.

'Liv, I need to talk to you.'

'Can't it wait until tomorrow?' she said, her voice uneven, slightly jerky. 'I've had a really rotten day, and—'

'I want to apologise,' he said quickly. 'What I said to you on Monday, about you treating me like a dogsbody. It was childish.'

'But understandable if me being your boss bothers you,' she said awkwardly.

'It doesn't bother me. Well, it doesn't now,' he added as her eyebrows rose, clearly questioning his remark. 'I've thought about it, and my reaction was stupid. You're the best person for this job, Liv.'

'I am?' she said, unable to hide her surprise, and he smiled a little ruefully.

'I couldn't do what you do. For a start I'd have decked half the staff in Admin by now.'

'I have to say I've been sorely tempted to do just that over the past week,' she declared.

'Yes, but you didn't,' he said gently, 'and that's why you're the boss, and I never will— or can—be.'

She smiled, and he smiled back, and there was so much heat in his eyes that her eyes skittered away, and she could feel her cheeks darkening, and her breath becoming ragged.

Oh, hell, she wanted him back. So much for all her talk about being an independent career-woman. She just wanted him back, holding her, loving her, but she couldn't ask him to return. A woman had her pride.

'Seth—'

'I owe you an even bigger apology for what I said about Phil,' he continued. 'What I said to you was cruel, and if I could turn back the clock, take back what I said—'

'I said a lot of things I shouldn't have,' she said, more than willing to meet him halfway. 'I guess... I guess the trouble is, we both have pretty quick tempers.'

'Well, I know that I do,' he said softly. 'But I would have said you were one of the sweetest-tempered women I know.'

Oh, to hell with pride, her mind whispered as her eyes met his. *Just ask him to come back. It's what you want, you know it is. Even if you can only have him back for a month, it will be enough, so ask him.*

'How...how are you getting on with Charlie?' she asked, opting for the softly-softly approach.

'The man's a Neanderthal.'

A splutter of laughter came from her. 'That's a bit rough, isn't it?'

'You're not living with him, Liv. All he ever thinks about is bedding women.'

'Don't most male doctors?' she observed, her brown eyes dancing.

'Maybe when they're twenty-three or twenty-four but, jeez, Liv, he's the same age as me. It's about time he grew up.'

'Right.' She nodded, and he had a very strong suspicion that she was laughing at him.

He could live with that. Her laughing at him was preferable to her being angry with him. It also meant that she might—just *might*—not jump down his throat if he suggested cooking dinner for her one night at her place.

'Liv—'

'There's a personal phone call for you, Olivia. Line 3—a Billy Norton,' Babs called from the bottom of the corridor. 'He says he needs to talk to you about somebody called George.'

'Who's Billy Norton?' Seth asked, as Olivia hurried back into her office and picked up the phone.

'A builder. The damp course in the house needs upgrading, and he came today to fix it. I left him in the house this morning, and—' She bit off the rest of what she'd been about to say as Billy's voice came down the line, sounding quite unlike his usual gruff, hearty self. 'What's wrong, Billy? One of my staff said it had something to do with George.'

'He's gone, Doctor. One minute he was there, watching what I was doing, and the next... I was positive I'd shut the front door, but... I've been out in the street whistling for him for the last two hours, calling his name, but there's just no sign of him.'

'Have you phoned the vet in case he's been taken there?' she said, shaking her head at Seth who was mouthing 'What's wrong?' at her.

'Doctor, I've phoned every vet in Glasgow but none of them have seen him, and neither have the police or the animal shelter people.'

'OK, what's wrong?' Seth asked the second she put down the phone.

'George has got out, and Billy can't find him,' she said, reaching for her coat and handbag. 'Seth, he's got no road sense. He's always on a lead unless he's in the park, and traffic terrifies him, and...' She clamped down on her lip to stop it from trembling, and shook her head. 'I know you must think I'm crazy—over-reacting—when George is just a dog—'

'George is *not* just a dog,' Seth interrupted. 'He's George, and you love him.'

She nodded, and swallowed hard. 'Could you let everyone in the department know where I've gone? I'll take my pager with me—'

'I'm coming with you. Liv, this is George,' he exclaimed as she gazed at him, startled. 'He may be a walking hearthrug, but he's your walking hearthrug, and...well, I've grown kind of fond of him, too.'

Tears filled her eyes, and she blinked them away furiously. Phil would never have volunteered to help look for George. Phil would have said good riddance to him.

'I... Thank you. I appreciate it,' she said with difficulty.

Billy Norton was pacing the street outside her house, looking harassed and upset.

'I just don't know how this could have happened,' he said the moment he saw them. 'I was sure the door was firmly shut, but—'

'Where have you looked?' she asked, cutting across his apology without compunction.

'In all the streets round the house, and in the park at the bottom of the road. He's not exactly

small and inconspicuous, so I was sure somebody would remember seeing him, but—'

'Maybe somebody took him in because they
knew you were at work,' Seth said firmly, seeing her lip tremble. 'Knowing George, he's
probably happily ensconced on somebody's
sofa, scoffing biscuits.'

She tried to smile. 'You're probably right,
but…it's starting to get dark, Seth, and if anything's happened to him—if somebody's taken
him away… He's my best friend. All the time
I was married to Phil he was always there for
me, and if he doesn't come back, if we don't
find him…'

'Liv, we *will* find him,' he said, putting his
arm round her and giving her a hug. 'Now, you
start knocking on doors and I'll check the streets
and the park again. If we split up, we'll cover
the area more quickly.'

He turned to go, and she put out her hand
quickly to stop him.

'I think he's looking for you,' she said, her
eyes shining with unshed tears. 'He's been missing you so badly ever since you left, and I
think—maybe in his doggy mind—he thought
that if he went out and looked for you…'

Seth's heart sank. He hoped to heaven George
wasn't looking for him. There were so many

roads in Glasgow, so much traffic. When he'd said this morning that he'd do anything to get back into Olivia's house again he hadn't meant this—he would never have meant this. If George really was gone... Unconsciously he shook his head. He refused to think like that, even for a second.

'We'll get him back, Liv.'

Two hours, Olivia thought as she trudged wearily back up Edmonton Road. She'd been searching for George for two hours and still there was no sign of him. She'd knocked on every door, called in on the local vet and at the police station, and everywhere the reply was the same. 'Sorry, Doctor, we haven't seen him.'

'I blame myself, Dr Mackenzie,' Billy declared, his face racked with guilt as she took her coat off and threw it over the settle in the hall. 'I know how much you love your dog.'

'It's OK, Billy,' she said as he packed up his toolbox, promising to be back first thing tomorrow. But it wasn't OK, and they both knew that it wasn't.

If only she knew what had happened it wouldn't be so bad, she realised as she walked slowly into the sitting room and sat down. It was the not knowing that was the hardest thing to bear. If he'd been knocked down and killed by a car she would have been devastated, but not knowing where he was, not knowing if somebody was hurting him...

Maybe she should go out again. Go down to the park, or try searching the warren of streets up behind the house again. Anything was better than sitting alone in the silent house. She had just got to her feet when she heard her front door open. It would be Seth. Seth returning to tell her that he hadn't found George. Seth returning to tell her that it was too dark now to go on searching and that they should wait until morning.

But he hadn't come back to tell her that. As she walked out of the sitting room and into the hall, the first thing she saw was George, looking wet, bedraggled and very woebegone. The second thing she saw was Seth's blinding smile.

'Where did you find him?' she gasped, her voice halfway between a laugh and a sob as she rushed forward to envelop George in a crushing hug. 'Where *was* he?'

'Well, I don't know where he's been since Billy discovered he'd gone, but I do know where he eventually ended up,' Seth replied. 'Morrison's Paint and DIY.'

'Morrison's...?'

'I was coming back up Edmonton Road, wondering how the hell I was going to tell you that I hadn't found him, when Ian Morrison hailed me from across the street. I thought he was going to ask me how I was getting on with the fireplace and, to be honest, I didn't want to stop, but he shouted that he had something belonging to you.'

'George?' She laughed, and Seth nodded.

'Apparently, Mr Morrison had gone through to his front shop to lock up before he began counting the day's takings, and he noticed George sitting outside so he took him in.'

'But where's he *been* all afternoon?' Olivia exclaimed as she draped a towel round George's shoulders and began to rub him dry.

'Who knows? All that matters is that he eventually had the sense to go to a place he knew.'

'It would be all those trips you made with him to the shop,' she said, as George wriggled free from her arms and padded through into the sitting room, looking for all the world like a medieval jousting horse with the towel trailing from his shoulders. 'He'd remember being there with you—remember the smell—and perhaps he thought you were still there.'

'That's what Mr Morrison figured, but frankly I don't care why he was there. I'm just so pleased we got him back.' For a moment Seth hovered uncertainly in the hall, then half turned. 'I'd better be going…'

'What do you mean, going?' she protested. 'You can't leave without having something to eat. You must be just as cold and wet as George. There's plenty of food in the fridge—'

'Chill-cook food?' he said with a hint of a smile, and she laughed.

'OK, so it's chill-cook food, but it will fill a space, and you must be starving.'

He was, he thought as he allowed her to take his jacket and accepted a towel to dry his hair, but not for food. He just wanted to be with her. Not even to make love to her, but just to be there with her, to be close to her, and to have her smile her wonderful smile at him again.

Take it slow, his mind reminded him. *You've blown this once already, so take it slow.*

And he did. All through dinner he kept the conversation light and frivolous, not mentioning Tony once, and it was she who brought up the subject of Charlie when they were washing the dishes.

'Is he really that bad a flatmate?' she asked, and without a moment's hesitation he happily slandered the dietetic technician.

'Liv, he's so bad I'm actually thinking of moving into hospital accommodation until my ceiling's fixed.'

She looked promisingly horrified. 'But, Seth, those flats are terrible. Concrete bunkers where you have to stand on the bed in order to open the wardrobe or you knock all your teeth out.'

'I know, but I can't stand living with Charlie for a minute longer,' he declared. 'He's driving me crazy.'

For a second she said nothing, and he held his breath. If she didn't offer what he was hoping she would offer, then he'd keep on wearing her down, working on her little by little, until he could prove to her that he really did love her. But if she did offer...

'You could move back in with me if you want,' she said, and he only just restrained himself from punching the air in triumph.

'Are you sure?' he said, schooling his expression with difficulty into one of uncertainty. 'I'd love to move back in—if you'll have me—but...'

The smile he had been hoping for suddenly lit up her face, taking his breath away. 'Of course I want you to move back in, you big ninny. George is missing you like crazy, and so am I.'

'Does that mean…?' Lord, he couldn't believe what he was hearing. 'When you say you've been missing me, does that mean…?'

'That one of the conditions of you moving back in is you have to sleep with the landlady?' She nodded. 'I'm afraid that's written into the contract.' He let out a whoop of delight, and she laughed as he tossed the dishcloth over his shoulder and pulled her into his arms. 'Seth, there's only one other condition you have to accept.'

'Name it, and it's yours,' he said.

'I don't want to hear any more talk of marriage.'

'Not a word,' he said solemnly. 'In fact,' he added, crossing his fingers behind his back, 'the "M" word is never going to pass my lips again.'

At least, not for a little while, he thought as she fell into his kiss and he revelled in her warmth, and heat, and fire. He'd wait a month—six weeks, tops—but somehow, some way, he was going to persuade this woman to marry him.

CHAPTER TEN

'WATSON FORRESTER will be back on Monday.'

'That should be interesting,' Olivia said through a mouthful of toothpaste.

'Are you really going to ask for his resignation the minute he walks through the door?' Seth asked as he stepped out of the shower and reached for a towel. 'I'm not saying he doesn't deserve it, but with Tony on suspension—and you and I both know he won't be coming back—is this really the best time for us to be losing another member of staff?'

'When was the last time Watson was an effective member of staff?' she said, putting her toothbrush back in the rack. 'I'm sorry, Seth, but I won't carry dead wood.'

He grinned as he towel-dried his hair. 'Olivia Mackenzie the Killer Clinical Director?'

'That's me.' She laughed. 'Mean, moody, magnificent.'

'I don't know about the mean and moody,' he said, reaching for her, 'but I'd definitely second the magnificent.' Quickly his fingers loosened the bath towel she'd wrapped round herself. 'For example, you have a magnificent set of curves down here, and you have an even more magnificent set of curves right up—'

'Work,' she interrupted. 'We have to go to work.'

'Spoilsport.' He grinned, planting a kiss on the top of her head. 'Do you think if we spoke nicely to Admin, they might rustle us up a relief doctor?'

She walked out of the bathroom and into her bedroom. 'I asked them that last week when I filed my report on Tony. They said they'd work on it.'

'In other words, don't hold your breath,' he sighed as he followed her. 'So, come what may, Watson gets the elbow on Monday.'

'Got it in one,' she said as she reached for her underwear. 'Do you think you might have time to pick up some groceries today? I'd do it myself, only—'

'No problem,' he replied, sitting down on the edge of the bed to better appreciate the view as she wriggled into her panties, then bent over to retrieve her trousers.

'Hey, stop ogling me,' she protested as she turned and saw him. 'You're making make me feel like a lap dancer.'

'Oh, good.' He grinned. 'Any chance of you coming over here and giving me a private performance?'

She shook her head at him. 'Behave, will you, and get yourself dressed.'

'I'd rather misbehave with you.'

She chuckled, her face bright and shining with happiness as she pulled her sweater over her head. 'So would I, but right now we have boring things to do like going to work and picking up groceries. I've made a list of what we need, but the most important thing is George's dog biscuits. He's down to the last one. I know he prefers human biscuits but... What?' she asked as Seth began to laugh. 'What's so funny about dog biscuits?'

'Nothing. I was just thinking how great this is, us living together, me picking up the groceries. We're just like—'

'Like what?' she said, her laughter disappearing, replaced by a look of deep suspicion

Red alert, red alert, his mind shrieked. *You almost said 'like a happily married couple'.*

'Like...like a couple who get on really well together,' he said quickly. 'Which we do, of course. In fact, we get on so well together that...' *Oh, even bigger mistake, Seth,* his mind protested as her eyes started to narrow. 'What I meant to say was—'

'Seth, if this is your not very subtle way of trying to raise the marriage question again—'

'The marriage question?' he repeated, opening his eyes very wide. 'Not me—never—uh-uh. The ''M'' word never crossed my mind for a second.'

'Good,' she said firmly, 'because you know what I said about that, and you know what you promised.'

He did, he thought morosely as he made them both breakfast, but why couldn't she get it through her thick skull that marriage wouldn't be the end of everything, but the beginning? OK, so they'd only been living together properly for a week, but...

'Whatever you do, don't blow it,' Jerry had warned him, 'because if you do, I don't think you'll get a third chance.'

Seth thought he wouldn't either as he and Olivia set off for the hospital, but it was getting really wearing having to constantly watch what he said. Dammit, he loved her, and he was pretty sure she loved him, but how on earth was he going to get her to admit it?

*   *   *

'Thank God it's Friday,' Jerry said with feeling. 'I don't know about the pair of you, but I think this week has seemed interminable.'

'You're lucky,' Seth said ruefully. 'At least you've got the weekend off. Olivia and I haven't.'

'Maybe you'll be lucky,' Jerry said. 'Today's been pretty quiet, so maybe you'll have a nice, peaceful—'

'Don't say it,' Olivia wailed. 'Don't tempt the gods. You know what happens the minute anybody tempts—' She came to a halt as the doors of the examination room opened and Madge from Reception appeared, ushering a harassed and dishevelled-looking young man and a heavily pregnant woman in front of her. 'Told you,' Olivia continued, throwing a withering glance in Jerry's direction. 'Never tempt fate.'

'We've a baby on the way here,' Madge exclaimed, 'and I don't think it's going to wait until Mrs Leadingham gets up to the labour ward.'

Olivia was at the young couple's side in an instant. 'OK, Madge. Phone Gideon Caldwell in Obs and Gynae and tell him we need him here p.d.q. Fiona...' She glanced round quickly. 'Where's Fiona?'

'Cubicle 3, suturing a knee wound,' Seth replied as he joined her. 'Looks like it's you and me for the delivery business.'

She had good cause to be grateful for his offer when Mrs Leadingham had clambered awkwardly up onto the trolley in cubicle 6 and they'd removed her underclothes. The baby's head was already crowning and the contractions were coming every minute.

'You were cutting this a bit fine, weren't you?' Seth smiled at Mr Leadingham who was gripping his wife's hand like a vice, his face white and anxious.

'We thought it was indigestion. The baby's not due until next week, you see, and—'

'I take it this is your first baby?' Olivia asked, using her left hand to control the rate of escape of the baby's head.

'And it's going to be our last,' Helen Leadingham groaned as another contraction ripped through her. 'Nobody told me it was going to hurt like this. If I'd known it was going to hurt like this, I'd have bought a dog instead.'

There was a small muscle twitching near the corner of Seth's mouth, and Olivia knew she daren't meet his eyes.

'Push, Helen,' she said encouragingly. 'Don't fight against the contractions, work with them.'

'That's…easy…for…you…to say,' the woman said breathlessly, her face turning scarlet as she pushed down hard, letting out a yell at the same time. 'You're…not…trying…to… deliver…a…truck.'

'Looks more like a sports car to me,' Seth observed as Olivia slipped the baby's cord over its head, then gently began to ease one of its shoulders free. 'Another couple of pushes, Helen. Just give us another couple of pushes and I guarantee you'll have your own custom-made Ferrari.'

Helen Leadingham gave a half-laugh, her face turned scarlet again and with a guttural cry she bore down. With a slide and a rush the baby shot out into Seth's hands.

'Is it a boy or a girl?' Mr Leadingham asked, hopping from one foot to the other, his face decidedly green.

'A girl,' Seth replied. 'You have a beautiful baby girl. Two arteries present in the cord?' he added under his breath, and Olivia nodded as she clamped it.

'Just the placenta to deliver,' she said, gently beginning to apply downward traction on the umbilical cord while she pressed equally gently on Mrs Leadingham's uterus to help the placenta on its way.

'Trying to make me redundant, are you, Seth?' Gideon Caldwell, the consultant from Obs and Gynae, asked as he emerged through the cubicle curtains with two of his staff.

'Not willingly, we can assure you.' Seth grinned. 'In fact, the only delivery we're really happy handling is pizza.'

'Perhaps,' the Obs and Gynae consultant declared as a small gush of blood came from Helen Leadingham, followed quickly by the placenta, 'but you've done a very good job.'

Mr Leadingham clearly thought so, too, as he gripped Seth's hand and shook it until Olivia thought he'd shake it off.

'I don't know what to say except thank you,' he exclaimed. 'I've never been so scared in all my life and...' The young man gulped, and blew his nose vigorously. 'Are you a father, Doctor?'

Seth shook his head. 'No, I'm not.'

'You should try it. I tell you...' He gazed down at his wife and daughter, and blew his nose again. 'Believe me, it's like nothing else in the world.'

Seth smiled, and his eyes met Olivia's over Mr Leadingham's head. Like an idiot, she smiled back.

What are you doing? her mind protested. *Look at him. He's got broodiness written all over him, and the last thing you want right now is a baby. OK, so maybe you're happier living with Seth than you'd ever have thought possible, but a baby would mean the end of your independence, and Seth might start talking about marriage again, and you don't want to get married, remember?*

But Baby Leadingham was seriously cute, she thought with a slight sigh as she watched Gideon place the little girl in the medi-crib. Cute and appealing, with her halo of golden curls, her little button nose and tiny rosebud lips. And it was thoughts like these that got a woman into serious trouble, Olivia realised wryly.

'Can I thank you, too, Doctor?' Helen said as one of their porters took hold of the end of her trolley and began wheeling her out of A and E. 'Frank's not much use in a crisis, and I'm ashamed to say I panicked a bit.'

'I think I would have panicked, too.' Olivia chuckled as Seth hurried off to help Fiona, who was struggling to support a very large man with an injured leg. 'I mean, there you were, expecting a nice controlled and supervised birth, and you end up in Accident and Emergency.'

Helen laughed. 'I suppose it will be something to tell my daughter when she grows up.

Would you thank your fiancé for me? I know Frank did, but I never got a chance to.'

'My fiancé…?'

'The nice doctor who was with you.' Helen coloured. 'Oh, dear, he's not your fiancé, is he? I'm so sorry. I just thought…the way he was looking at you…'

'It's all right, Helen,' Olivia said hurriedly. 'It was an easy mistake to make.'

Which was a really stupid thing to say, she thought with a groan as Helen was wheeled away. How was it an easy mistake to make? Had Seth somehow secretly branded her over the past week with the words, 'Under Offer'?

Jerry was just as bad, she thought irritably as she watched the specialist registrar shoot across the examination room towards cubicle 1. The minute he'd discovered Seth was living with her again she could tell from his expression that he was mentally making arrangements for the wedding and starting work on his best man speech.

Why couldn't everyone accept that she was happy as she was—that she didn't want a piece of paper and a ring on her finger? Seth had never said he loved her, and she didn't expect him to. Eventually she knew that he'd get bored playing couples and then he'd walk, and it would be so much easier if all he had to do was pack a suitcase.

And what about you? her heart whispered as she walked out of the examination room and headed for her office. Will it be easier for you when he walks away with only a suitcase?

I'm not going to think about that, she told the annoying little voice. *Right now Seth and I are having fun, and that's all I'm going to think about.*

'*There* you are,' Babs exclaimed with relief as she hurried down the corridor towards Olivia, clutching a trauma pack. 'Massive pile-up on the M8. Eight cars, three lorries and a motor-cyclist. The ambulances from the Merkland Memorial are already there and they're expecting staff from the Hillhead General, but they need every doctor they can get.'

'Have you alerted our ambulance crew?' Olivia asked, slipping off her white coat and thanking her lucky stars she'd decided to wear trousers that morning.

'They're on their way,' Babs replied, opening the door of their equipment cupboard and pulling out an orange flying suit, 'but the police say they need help urgently so they've called out the air ambulance. The helicopter should be landing on the roof in five minutes to pick up you and Seth.'

Olivia felt her stomach heave as she stared at the suit. She hated helicopters. The first time she'd flown in one she'd thrown up all over the paramedic, and the second time she'd been airborne she'd thrown up all over the pilot.

'Is there something wrong?'

Babs's gaze was fixed on her, curious, bewildered, and Olivia managed to smile as she wriggled into the flying suit and zipped it up.

'Not a thing,' she declared. 'Where's Seth?'

'He's already on his way to the roof.'

He would be, Olivia thought grimly. He was probably one of those awful gung-ho types with a secret yearning to hold a pilot's licence.

He was.

'Mac and I have flown together quite a few times,' Seth shouted over the whirr of the helicopter's rotor blades as they took off from the roof of the Belfield, 'and I'm always telling him that if he ever wants to swap jobs with me he only has to say the word. There's nothing I'd like better than to fly one of these babies.'

The pilot said something Olivia didn't catch, but before she could ask him to repeat it he suddenly steered the helicopter into a sharp, stomach-churning left bank and she ceased to care what his answer had been.

'Of course I wouldn't get bored,' Seth declared as the paramedic sitting next to him said something. 'How could I possibly get bored? Being up here every day, dipping and hovering, wheeling and diving—'

'Seth, shut up.'

He glanced across at her, puzzled, and so did the paramedic whose identity tag proclaimed him to be Donnie MacLeod. 'Wouldn't you like to fly in one of these every day? Liv, it's the closest thing to being a bird. Being up here in the thermals, swooping and diving—'

'Seth, if you don't stop talking about swooping and diving you're shortly going to be seeing the eggs and bacon you so lovingly cooked for me this morning coming back to you in a rather unappetising way.'

His jaw dropped. 'You're *scared?*'

'Yes, I'm scared,' she said through clenched teeth. 'I *hate* helicopters.'

'But—'

'But nothing, Seth. Just *shut up.*'

'Better do as your wife says,' Mac shouted over his shoulder, and Donnie grinned and Olivia shut her eyes and counted to ten.

What was it with everybody today? First it had been Mrs Leadingham thinking Seth was her fiancé, and now the pilot and paramedic thought she was his wife. She was not his wife. She was never going to be his wife, and if her stomach would just settle down, and she could get out of this damned helicopter, she'd tell him so.

'I can see the ambulances from the Merkland, but there's no sign of any from the Hillhead General,' Seth observed after they'd been in the air for what to Olivia felt like an eternity but what probably was, in reality, no more than ten minutes.

Olivia risked a quick glance out of the helicopter window, but all she could think was that if it looked so bad from up here it must be even worse on the ground.

It was.

'Messy,' Seth murmured as he jumped out of the helicopter, and she and Donnie followed him.

Carnage would have been a more accurate word, Olivia thought as she stared at the scene in front of her. The eight cars, three lorries and motorcyclist had ploughed straight into one another, sending broken glass and twisted metal across the motorway. Now an eerie, unnatural silence hung over everything. A silence that was broken only by the occasional squeal and scrape of collapsing metal, and the ominous smell of petrol and diesel fumes.

If this lot caught fire…

'They never learn, do they, Docs?' a policemen said bitterly as he joined them. 'It's been foggy all morning—visibility down to fifty metres—and yet they drive like it was a beautiful summer's day, sitting on one another's bumpers, never thinking what they're going to do if somebody has to suddenly brake sharply.'

Some of them would never brake again, Olivia thought as she watched the paramedics from the Merkland Memorial carry two body bags past.

'Has anybody started triage?' she asked as they followed the policeman across the motorway, gingerly skirting the broken glass and puddles which weren't rain water but leaking petrol.

'Doc Taylor from the Merkland is co-ordinating everything.' The policeman pointed to a tall bespectacled man talking to one of the firemen. 'I think he'll be glad of your help.'

He was, and his face lit up when he saw Seth.

'Well, if this doesn't beat all—old do-or-die-Hardcastle. Still practising medicine, are you,

Seth? I'd have thought they'd have rumbled you years ago.'

'Nope, I'm still getting away with it.' Seth grinned. 'This is ''Vulture'' Taylor, Liv,' he continued as she glanced from him to Dr Taylor in obvious confusion. 'Known in ambulance circles as Vulture because he always turns up at the scene of big disasters. He and I have been in some pretty tight corners over the years, but we've always managed to live to tell the tale, haven't we, Vulture?'

Dr Taylor laughed, and Olivia managed a small smile in return.

What was it with men? The slightest whiff of danger and, instead of behaving sensibly, they came over all macho and John Wayne.

'What's the situation?' she asked pointedly, and Dr Taylor dug a notebook out of his pocket.

'We've two fatalities so far, four walking wounded and the rest are major chest and leg injuries. We were hoping the Hillhead mob might have got here by now, but...' He sighed and shrugged. 'The most urgent cases still in need of treatment are the motorcyclist and one of the car drivers. I've got a fireman giving the motorcyclist basic first aid, but we can't risk sending anyone in to treat the car driver until the fire crew stabilise the lorry that crashed into him. They're working on that now.'

Olivia could see what he meant. The articulated lorry in question was lying precariously on top of the car while its load was balanced awkwardly on the motorway verge. If it moved just an inch...

'Liv, you and Donnie take the motorcyclist,' Seth declared. 'I'll take the car driver.'

Why am I not surprised? she thought irritably. Well, if old 'do-or-die' Hardcastle was itching to be in the thick of things, so be it.

'Fine,' she said, and without a backward glance she and Donnie headed over to the motorcyclist.

'His name's Allan Stewart,' the fireman declared, relinquishing his position beside the motorcyclist with clear relief. 'Glasgow coma scale 15. I immobilised his neck, and I've been giving him oxygen through a re-breathing mask, but I haven't been able to do much else.'

'You've done exactly what you should.' Olivia smiled as Donnie set up his portable monitor. 'Do you know what happened to him? It could help me in his examination.'

'He hit that car over there at 110 kilometres an hour, and was thrown 20 metres across the road.'

Olivia winced. 'He's lucky to be alive.'

'The car driver wasn't so lucky,' the fireman replied, and Olivia swallowed hard.

'Could you stay with us in case I need a third pair of hands?' she asked, and the fireman nodded.

'Not much I can do anywhere else at the moment. We've cut a hole to let your colleague get into the car that's under the lorry, and until he reports back on what state the driver's in, we wait.'

She glanced over her shoulder quickly as the lorry in question gave an ominous groan. 'It *is* quite safe under there, though, isn't it?' she asked uncertainly, and the fireman grinned.

'Nope, but that's all part of the fun of the job.'

The fun of the job? Right. Seth was underneath that lorry, attending to the car driver, and this was *fun?*

'Doctor…?'

Donnie was gazing at her pointedly, and she pulled herself together. This was no time to start worrying. Seth knew what he was doing. He wouldn't take unnecessary risks.

Yes, he would, a little voice whispered at the back of her head, but there was nothing she could do about it. Not when she had a patient who needed her.

'Trachea central, but his chest expansion is poor and he's hardly shifting any air,' she murmured, as she sounded the motorcyclist's chest. 'I'm guessing multiple rib fractures on the right side,' she added as she gently felt the young man's chest and heard him groan. 'But there's also a section of his chest wall moving paradoxically.'

'Flail chest?' Donnie said as he set up an IV line, and she nodded.

'That's what I think. We need to perform an oral intubation.'

With the fireman holding the motorcyclist's head firmly, she quickly loosened the hard collar he'd placed round the young man's neck then, as Donnie oxygenated him with a bag mask, she applied cricoid pressure and slipped a tracheal tube down his throat.

'The tube's in, Doc,' Donnie said after he'd checked the ventilation with his stethoscope. 'Good bilateral breath sounds. You can release your cricoid pressure now.'

She did, but though the young man's breathing improved immediately his blood pressure remained stubbornly low.

'Internal haemorrhage?' Donnie suggested as he set up another IV line.

It was a distinct possibility, Olivia thought, but before she could say so she had to duck quickly as a car exploded and the back wheel of the motorcycle that had crashed into it suddenly flew through the air.

Her eyes met the fireman's. 'Yes, I know. This is all part of the fun of the job, but could you perhaps arrange for there to be a little less fun and some more peace and quiet?'

He grinned back at her. 'I'll do my best, Doc, but I can't guarantee it. I wonder how your colleague's getting on?'

Olivia wondered, too, but tried not to think about it.

Gently she rocked the motorcyclist's hips. The young man's pelvis felt grossly unstable, which suggested that a large amount of blood was collecting there.

'Ringer's lactate,' she ordered, and as Donnie ran it into the young man as fast as the two IV lines would allow, she began wrapping a large, wide bandage corset-like round the motorcyclist's pelvis to stabilise it.

'There's not much more we can do here,' Donnie murmured once she'd finished.

There wasn't. What the young man needed now was the operating theatre, and as though he'd read her thoughts Dr Taylor appeared.

'Is he ready to go?' he asked as Donnie placed a warming blanket round the motorcyclist.

'We just need to immobilise his spine before we transfer him to the scoop stretcher,' Olivia replied.

Dr Taylor nodded. 'Do you want to go with him in the ambulance, or would you rather wait for Seth? The Hillhead mob have finally arrived—late as usual—and we may as well give them something to do, unless you have any objections.'

'None at all.' She laughed, only for her laughter to die in her throat as she got to her feet.

From across the motorway there came a shuddering groan, followed by the dreadful sound of splintering metal, and as she turned quickly in its direction she saw the props supporting the lorry suddenly give way. For an agonising second the lorry hung suspended, and then with a crash it collapsed on top of the car, and her heart stopped.

Dimly she heard Dr Taylor's horrified oath, but she couldn't say anything. All she could think was that Seth had been underneath that lorry. He'd been treating the car driver, and now he was dead. He couldn't have survived that—nobody could have survived that—and her legs gave way as a shaft of pain twisted through her and she sat down hard on the cold, glass-covered ground.

He was dead, and she was never going to be able to hold him in her arms again. Dead, and she would never again hear his laugh or see his eyes light up when he looked at her. Dead, and she was never going to be able to tell him how much she loved him—and she did love him—but now he would never know that because in the space of a second her whole world had gone.

With a cry of anguish she put her head on her knees. Why hadn't she told him how she felt? The last word she'd spoken to him had been a curt 'Fine', and now there was never going to be a chance to say anything else.

Vaguely she became aware that somebody had crouched down beside her, and she lifted her head to see one of the firemen gazing at her with concern.

'He's dead, isn't he?' she whispered, her eyes huge and strained.

'His leg is broken, and he's got massive chest injuries, but considering he was in a major pile-up I'd say that driver is one very lucky man.'

'I don't mean the car driver,' she said harshly. 'I meant Seth. Dr Hardcastle.'

The fireman smiled. 'Of course he's not dead. Nine lives has old do-or-die Seth. He'll probably have a heck of a sore shoulder tomorrow, but we got him and the car driver out just before the lorry toppled, and he's fine.'

'Fine?' she repeated faintly, not believing him. She glanced across to the shattered car. Nobody could walk away from a wreck like that. Nobody. She cleared her throat. 'You don't have to lie to me. I can take the truth.'

'Doctor—'

'Hey, sweetheart, what's wrong?'

Her head snapped round at the sound of the familiar voice, and she looked up to see a pair of sparkling blue eyes grinning down at her. Her mouth worked soundlessly for a second, and then she burst into tears. 'I thought you were *dead!*'

'Nah, not me,' Seth declared, taking her hands and pulling her to her feet. 'Mr Invincible, that's me.'

'Don't *ever* do that to me again,' she sobbed. 'When I thought you were squashed under that lorry, and I pictured my life without you… Seth, it was awful. Grey, and empty, and lonely... So very, very lonely.'

'Hey, I'm here, I'm OK,' he insisted, gathering her to his chest. 'Nothing is ever going to happen to me.'

'But it might,' she cried, her voice muffled by his orange flying suit. 'And if you weren't here...if I lost you...'

'Liv, you are *not* going to lose me,' he said, tightening his hold on her. 'I'm here for the duration. Hell, you couldn't get rid of me even if you wanted to.'

She gave a hiccuping laugh. 'I don't want to get rid of you.'

'And that's why I think we should get married,' he declared. 'Yes, I know you don't want to marry me,' he added as she tried to interrupt, 'but, Liv, we're the perfect couple.'

She pulled a handkerchief out of her flying suit pocket, and blew her nose. 'Why?'

He looked startled. 'Well, George likes me for a start. He doesn't bark or growl at me—'

'Seth, George likes everybody, even the postman.'

He frowned. 'OK, how about the fact that we're great together in bed. That's got to be a plus, hasn't it?'

'A plus, yes,' she agreed, 'but great sex isn't a good enough reason for two people to get married. What's going to happen when we're too old to have sex?'

'Liv, we're never going be too old to have sex. I'll be making love to you when we're ninety.'

'We won't both be ninety,' she pointed out. 'When I'm ninety, you'll be ninety-two.'

He stared heavenwards with exasperation. 'All right, dammit, how about I love you? I can't imagine my life without you. I don't *want* to imagine my life without you.'

She blinked. 'You love me? You actually love me?'

'Haven't I been saying so for the last ten minutes?' he protested, and she shook her head.

'You said that you and George have bonded, and that we're great in bed. You never said you loved me.'

He dug his hands into his pockets. 'Well, I do. I never thought I'd ever hear myself saying that to a woman, but...Liv, you mean everything to me. You're my sunshine, the bright jewel in my life that makes everything worthwhile.'

Tears filled her eyes again, and began trickling down her cheeks. 'I love you, too.'

'You do?' he exclaimed. 'Then for crying out loud, why didn't you say so?'

'I didn't know before,' she said. 'I didn't know until I thought I'd lost you, that I never see you again, and... I don't ever want to feel that way again.'

'So, are you going to marry me, and we can live happily ever after, me doing DIY, you baking in the kitchen—?'

'*You* doing DIY?' she exclaimed, her eyebrows raised, and he grinned.

'OK—OK, I'll rephrase that. Are you going to marry me, so we can live happily ever after, you doing the DIY and me baking in the kitchen? Olivia, I want us to get married,' he continued. 'I want to take hundreds of photographs of little Tristram and Isolde and bore the pants off Jerry.'

'Seth, those are lousy names for kids.'

'We can argue about that when they arrive,' he said dismissively. 'Are you going to marry me?'

'We don't need to get married for me to have your children,' she pointed out, and he sighed.

'Yes, we do. I'm an old-fashioned guy, and I think I should be married to the mother of my kids. And you'll make my mother so happy. She's all but given up on me ever getting married, and you wouldn't deprive a little old lady of the chance of happiness, would you?'

She gazed at him suspiciously. 'How old is your mother?'

'Sixty-two. OK, so she's not a little old lady,' he said as Olivia rolled her eyes, 'and she'd probably kill me if she ever heard me describing her as one, but it's her dearest wish to see me walking up the aisle, and I'm getting desperate here.'

'You want a church wedding?' she said in surprise, and he looked rueful.

'Liv, my family have been desperate to get me hitched for years. You think they're going to settle for anything less?'

'Deb wouldn't either,' she murmured. 'You should have seen her face when Phil and I got married in a registry office.'

'Is that a yes?' he demanded. 'Are you going to marry me?'

She sighed. 'I wanted to be an independent career-woman.'

He reached out and cupped her face in his hands, his eyes dark and tender and so full of love that she felt her breath catch in her throat.

'Liv, you still can be. I don't want to be your jailer. I just want to hold you, and to keep you, and to love you until the end of time.'

'Oh, Seth,' she whispered through a throat so tight it hurt. 'That's the nicest thing anybody's ever said to me.'

'So are you going to marry me?' he asked, and when she nodded he punched the air in triumph. 'About damn time.'

He gathered her into his arms and kissed her, and when she finally surfaced, laughing and gasping for air, she saw Dr Taylor watching them.

'I hate to break this up,' he said, the corners of his mouth twitching slightly, 'but I really think I should point out that both of you have a hospital to go back to, and unless you move pretty sharpish you're undoubtedly going to be flattened by the salvage team.'

'We're sorry,' Olivia began hurriedly.

Seth said, 'No, we're not.'

'Sounds like the two of you are going to have an interesting marriage,' Dr Taylor observed.

'Are you going back in the helicopter or the road ambulance?'

'The road ambulance,' Olivia said firmly.

At the same moment Seth said, 'The helicopter.'

'Like, I said.' Dr Taylor grinned. 'A very interesting marriage.'

And as Olivia stared up at Seth and saw the love in his eyes as he gazed back at her, she knew Dr Taylor was right.

MEDICAL ROMANCE™

Large Print

Titles for the next six months…

April

DOCTOR AND PROTECTOR	Meredith Webber
DIAGNOSIS: AMNESIA	Lucy Clark
THE REGISTRAR'S CONVENIENT WIFE	Kate Hardy
THE SURGEON'S FAMILY WISH	Abigail Gordon

May

THE POLICE DOCTOR'S SECRET	Marion Lennox
THE RECOVERY ASSIGNMENT	Alison Roberts
ONE NIGHT IN EMERGENCY	Carol Marinelli
CARING FOR HIS BABIES	Lilian Darcy

June

ASSIGNMENT: CHRISTMAS	Caroline Anderson
THE POLICE DOCTOR'S DISCOVERY	Laura MacDonald
THE MIDWIFE'S NEW YEAR WISH	Jennifer Taylor
A DOCTOR TO COME HOME TO	Gill Sanderson

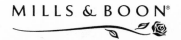

MILLS & BOON®

Live the emotion

0305 LP 2P P1 Medical

MEDICAL ROMANCE™

Large Print

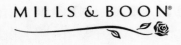

MILLS & BOON®

Live the emotion

0305 LP 2P P2 Medical